D1192253

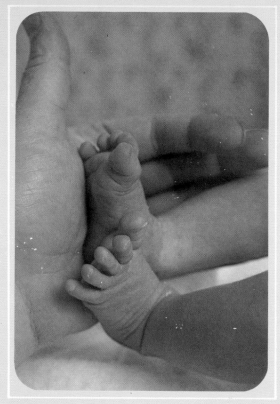

THE HOME BIRTH BOOK

BY CHARLOTTE AND FRED WARD
INTRODUCTION BY ASHLEY MONTAGU, Ph. D.

THE
HOME
BIRTH
BOOK

There was a child went forth every day;
And the first object he look'd upon, that object he became;
And that object became part of him for the day, or a certain
part of the day, or for many years, or stretching cycles
of years.

His own parents,
He that father'd him, and she that had conceiv'd him in
her womb, and birth'd him,
They gave this child more of themselves than that;
They gave him afterward every day—they became part of him.

THERE WAS A CHILD WENT FORTH
Walt Whitman

PHOTO BY CHARLOTTE WARD

THE HOME BIRTH BOOK

Charlotte and Fred Ward

Contributors: James D. Brew, M.D. • Nancy Mills •
Russell J. Bunai, M.D. • Miriam Kelty, Ph.D. •
Edward Kelty, Ph.D. • Lester R. Hazell • Patricia Nicholas •
Raven Lang • Tonya Brooks • Janet L. Epstein, C.N.M., M.S.M. •
Marion McCartney, C.N.M., B.S.N. • Esther Herman • Fran Ventre

Photographs by
Fred Ward

Introduction by
Ashley Montagu, Ph.D.

Edited by
Roger Glenn Brown

Designed by
Thomas R. Smith

An INSCAPE Book

Dolphin Books
Doubleday & Company, Inc.
Garden City, New York
1977

Dolphin Books Edition: 1977
Original version published by Inscape Publishers/Washington, D.C.
International Standard Book Number: 0-385-12559-3
Library of Congress Catalog No.: 76-40642
Copyright ©1976, 1977 by Charlotte Ward and Fred Ward
Copyright ©1976, by Ashley Montagu
Printed in the United States of America
All Rights Reserved

contents

DEDICATION

Our book on home birth was truly a "labor of love." It is with this same feeling of love that we dedicate it to our parents—Alberta and J Mayes and Bess and Newman Ward—and to our children—Kim, Chris, and Laura. Two small groups, perhaps, but without either, there would have been no book and no real comprehension of what childbirth at home really means.

C. W.

F. W.

ACKNOWLEDGMENTS

We sincerely appreciate the assistance and encouragement of those who shared their information and ideas with us.

Especially meaningful to us was the work of Regina Greenspun, who graciously gave of her time and talents.

We look back with affection to our early experiences with dear friends in La Leche League who had similar philosophies and offered continuous support through the years: Judy Melson, who inspired us with her own home birth story; Joan Conklin; Lee Bernheisel; Joan Marie Segreti; Jean Bonde, R.N.; and Richard Applebaum, M.D.

We feel a special bond with Mikie Donohue, R.N., and Ritva Hackel, R.N., who helped bring Christopher into the world; and with Janet Epstein, R.N., who coached Laura's birth; and with Maureen and Tara Van Emmerik; Dessa Gray, and Lucy Wise who celebrated with us.

Our thanks go to our friends Howertine Duncan, at the National Medical Library; Betty Dalsemer; Doris Waldbaum, Ph.D.; and Pilar Farnsworth of BIRTH, all of whom made significant research suggestions.

We greatly appreciate those who gave of their time and expertise: Julie Boruff of American Society for Psychoprophylaxis in Obstetrics; Doris Haire, Past-President of International Childbirth Education Association; Cecelia Chaney of Parent and Child; Pat Bealle of La Leche League; Bev Eanes, R.N.; Helen Browne, Director of Frontier Nursing Service; Helen Hoffman of Chicago Maternity Center; Tina Long of H.O.M.E.; Kate Bowland of the Birth Center; Nancy Mulver, R.N., of Howard University; Susan Doering of Johns Hopkins University; Janet Gruwell of the Oregon Historical Society; Amy Kesselman of the Washington County, Oregon, Historical Museum; Mary Hilliard, R.N., of the University of Florida; James Minard, Ph.D., of New Jersey Medical School; and Laura Wilson of the World Health Organization.

introduction

Should Babies Be Born at Home?

By Ashley Montagu

Should babies be born at home? What a question! Where else should they be born, if not in the home? The hospital? But I had thought that a hospital was a place where one went for relief from sickness or injury. I would not have thought, had I not known it to be the fact, that the most important event in the life of a family, the birth of a child, was best celebrated away from the home, away from the family, in a hospital—in a hospital to which the sick and the injured go. Is pregnancy a sickness? Is the birth of a child a disease? Is the arrival of a new baby something in which the rest of the family should not share? Is it bad for the mother, or for anyone else, if birth takes place in the home?

Most persons over sixty were probably born at home. I was, and so were most of my friends. The vast majority of human beings alive at this moment were born at home, and the vast majority of births in the world taking place at this moment are occurring in the home. In the greater part of Europe most births still take place in the home. How, then, does it come about that in the United States the greater number of births take place in the hospital? In the larger cities of this country well over 90 percent of the births take place in the hospital.

The history of this development will not long detain us. It is largely the doing of the medical profession. To our doctors we probably owe as much, if not more than, to any other profession for the all-round general improvement in the health of Americans, the virtual elimination of many diseases, the reduction in the virulence of others, decreased maternal and infant mortality rates, and the increase in longevity. The average American male may expect to live to be sixty-nine years of age, the average American female may expect to live to seventy-five—almost exactly double the expectation of life one hundred years ago. All this is largely the doing of the medical profession. But somehow this progress has been achieved at the cost of an increasing specialization and mechanization of the practice of medicine. The much esteemed old family doctor, the general practitioner, over the course of the years got to know his family and his patients so intimately that he couldn't but help treating them as human beings. Today the horse-and-buggy doctor has been replaced by a specialist who is an authority on either the right or the left nostril, but not on both, and to whom the patient is a set of symptoms to which a body happens to be attached. Many doctors seem to have forgotten that the care of the patient begins with caring for the patient. The general idea seems to be to treat as many patients as possible. This tendency results in an arrangement whereby if the doctor can persuade his patients to go to a particular hospital he can see them all there without the necessity of having to run all over the place, and as a consequence see fewer patients than he could by this arrangement. Furthermore, the hospital offers the doctor relief from many obligations which he would otherwise have to carry out himself; a good deal of the drudgery associated with the practice of medicine is taken over by the hospital. This is particularly the case where birth is concerned.

One can readily understand and sympathize with the physician's desire to have his patients in the hospital for the delivery of their babies. It is a great convenience for the doctor, but is it good for anyone else? Is it, eventually, good for the doctor himself? Is it good for the baby, for the mother, for society? The answer to all these questions is in the negative. In fact, the present heavy burden on doctors could be relieved by relying more heavily on trained nurses or

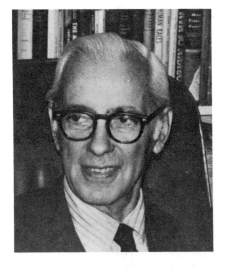

Ashley Montagu is the author of numerous books includng the best seller, Touching. *He has long been a proponent of prepared childbirth and childbirth at home, and has been a moving force behind the International Childbirth Education Association.*

midwives in home delivery situations. The health of babies would be enhanced because they would not be exposed to many of the diseases common in hospitals and because they would begin life in an alert and unmedicated state. Mothers would benefit because they would bring new life into the world with the support and comfort of husbands and other family loved ones. And finally, our society would reap a rich harvest because future generations would be composed of people who begin life in a more human way.

Children should be born in the home in which they are going to live and of which they are going to form a part. The objections to hospitalization for childbirth are many, the most important of them all being that the hospital tends to dehumanize the mother-child relationship, the very relationship out of which all humanity grows.

The child, in most hospitals—in spite of the advent of rooming-in—is separated from the mother, and the mother from the child *when they most need each other*. Mother and child most need each other during the first forty-eight hours after birth. Let me explain why.

From the standpoint of the newborn who, during the process of getting born has received an enormous number of new stimulations quite unlike those which it experienced during its development in the peaceful environment of the womb, getting born is a comparatively rough experience. The newborn is called upon to make all sorts of adjustments to the new environment into which it is thrust. It must breathe in oxygenated air, its lungs must begin to function, the heart must adapt itself both in position and in function to the new demands which are made upon it, and so on. At this time, more than at any other in its life, it requires every reassurance that all is well and there is promise of good things to come. And this is the very time we choose to separate it from the one person in the world who can give it that reassurance and promise. What the baby needs is the caress of its mother's body and the reassurance which being put to nurse at her breast gives it.

The mother needs the baby almost as much as the baby needs her. The mother is dependent very largely upon the undisturbed relationship with her baby for her own welfare.

Let this be underscored with the facts. When the baby is put to nurse at the mother's breast shortly after birth, not only is the breast stimulated to begin functioning, but three great obstetrical problems are in most cases solved virtually at once. These are the postpartum hemorrhage, the beginning of the return of the uterus to normal size, and the completion of the third stage of labor, which is the detachment and ejection of the placenta.

In most hospitals the mother is deprived of these benefits, whereas in the home she would be likely to enjoy them. In addition to these psysiological benefits there are, of course, the added psychological benefits which accrue both to her and to the baby. The continuity of the relationship between mother and baby should not under normal conditions ever be disturbed. Yet from the moment of birth this relationship is progressively disturbed in the hospital. The routinized procedures of the hospital interfere with the development of the natural functions of both mother and baby. As Professor Harry and Ruth Bakwin point out, "The obstetrical hospital is in good part responsible 'for the failure of many mothers to breast-feed their babies." More often than not no effort is made to initiate breast-feeding, but instead a bottle formula is prescribed for the baby, and since this satisfies the baby's appetite, the baby

3

is discouraged from sucking at the breast, and the stimulus for the secretion of milk is thus effectively removed. A hard glass or plastic lukewarm bottle with a rubber tire at the end of it is not a desirable substitute for the mother's breast.

The feeding demands of the baby do not function by the clock. Yet the practice of bringing the baby to the mother at fixed times and for limited periods, as is done in the hospital, does violence both to the mother's and the baby's needs. We seem to have a genius for starting off on the wrong foot from the moment the human being is born. As for the formula or cow's milk contained in that bottle, it should not be fed to babies because it contains the wrong quantities of fats and proteins and is hard on the baby's metabolic system. Furthermore, bottle feeding deprives the infant of experiences at the breast fundamental for its healthy mental as well as physical development.*

The birth of a new member of the family should be a family matter, not a series of problems for comparatively uninterested strangers in the psychologically impersonal environment of the hospital. The father of the child to be born should be a partner in the process of birth. He should be with the mother throughout the experience. It is at this time that the firmest psychological bonds between husband and wife are established. As a result of joining in the birth experience *together* each grows to mean more to the other and to their children than could be accomplished by any other means. It is during this period that the wife falls most profoundly in love with her husband, and the husband becomes more deeply involved in his wife and in his family. Instead, under prevailing conditions, the husband is not permitted to share in the experience, but must wait nervously and

*See Ashley Montagu, *Touching*. New York, Columbia University Press, 1971.

expectantly far removed from the one who most needs him. The wife too is often left alone, or in the charge of a nurse who is busily occupied somewhere else and occasionally pops her head in to see that things are "all right," or maybe in the presence of a strange young intern, or else holding the hand of her obstetrician upon whom she projects all the love she has to give, and which should properly be received by her husband—and returned by him. At home the husband would be where he belongs, with his wife, and no one should dare keep these two asunder at this most important period in their lives. With the increasing number of "natural childbirths" we have abundant and increasing evidence of the importance and value of the presence of the husbands during the birth process. The presence of one husband outweighs in value all the sedatives and medications in the world.

If there are any other children in the family they should also be made part of the household that is expecting the new brother or sister. They can accompany mother to the visits with the obstetrician and be present at all the examinations, and they can be present at the birth of their new sibling. This will all depend upon the parents' feelings in these matters. Some may feel that they need not be present at the birth itself, in which case the children should be fully prepared as early as possible, and encouraged to anticipate with all the pleasure possible the new addition to the family. Long before the new baby arrives is the time to anticipate any difficulties which might arise out of sibling rivalry. If the children are properly prepared and made to feel that their bonds with their family will be strengthened by the arrival of the new baby rather than weakened, much heartache will be avoided. As soon as feasible the other children should be introduced to their new sibling, while the new arrival is nursing at his mother's breast.

Under present conditions, when mother goes to the hospital the creature considered responsible for this dastardly separation is the new baby. No wonder the children abandoned at home want to strangle him or gouge his eyes out. For small children this is a much worse experience than it would be for a woman whose husband suddenly appeared, after an appreciable absence, with a beautiful young thing and then announced to his wife, "Mary, this is Gloria, my new co-wife. She will live together with us hereafter and I hope we will all have a jolly good time." It might be less of a shock to some wives than the experience of having the new baby introduced into the household without so much as a by-your-leave is to many children.

The family is a unit, and its unity should never be broken. If that unity must be disturbed it should never be in the manner so customarily and mechanically produced by the obstetrical hospital.

Should babies be born at home? Of course they should, for that is where they belong.

Happily, just as the return to breast-feeding—initiated entirely by women mainly under the auspices of La Leche League—is now gaining momentum, so there is a new movement advocating a return to childbirth at home.*

This book is a symbol of that movement. Its inspiring text and magnificent photographs should prove extremely encouraging to those young couples who are contemplating the rewarding experience of home childbirth.

*See "The Association for Childbirth at Home," below, p. 143.

part 1

The
Personal
Dimension

By Charlotte Ward

Charlotte's Story

Birth is a matter of heart. Although the experience of childbirth is unique to each woman with each labor, characteristic sensations accompany one stage, and then the next, until the baby forcefully emerges. A woman's body may not register all of these typical vibrations as they pulse through her, but the emotional quality of her birth-giving will be with her always. This indelible record affects the physical progress of her present laboring and all future births as well as her relationships with her family and all future children. Continually rewarding is childbirth remembered with joy.

How to achieve such a birth?—when each woman experiences the physical process uniquely; when each woman exists in different circumstances; when each woman perceives life from a distinct point of view; in short, when each woman is an *individual*? The simple answer: by having the baby at home. Among the people whom she loves and who love her best, she can be at ease. Those most suited to meet her needs are her own family.

The home and the family are integral. In the home, birth becomes a means to an end, not an end in itself. Home birth means continuity: there is a natural progression from caring between man and woman to caring between parent and child. In the home, individuals find self-expression; hospitals, on the other hand, operate by rules, generalizations, expertise, diversity, objectivity, decentralization, machinery, efficiency. Hospitals cannot *care* as can the family in the home.

Given a normal pregnancy, merely "delivering" a live baby is all but inevitable. What matters is that each baby be "born" in a healthful and considerate way so that the family looks upon his coming with love, so that he perceives his new wider environment as loving. Home birth signifies the family lovingly joining hands to welcome an expansion of their own group.

At home, the mother is assured of familiar territory. Her emotions are supported and her spirit freed to concentrate on priorities: herself and her coming child. Her family stands as her strength. Their approval nourishes her ability to enjoy childbirth; their presence gives her courage to be truly human. Home birth remains one of the great celebrations of family—the endless connection.

Throughout her pregnancy Charlotte continued a close relationship with three-year-old Kim, her first-born.

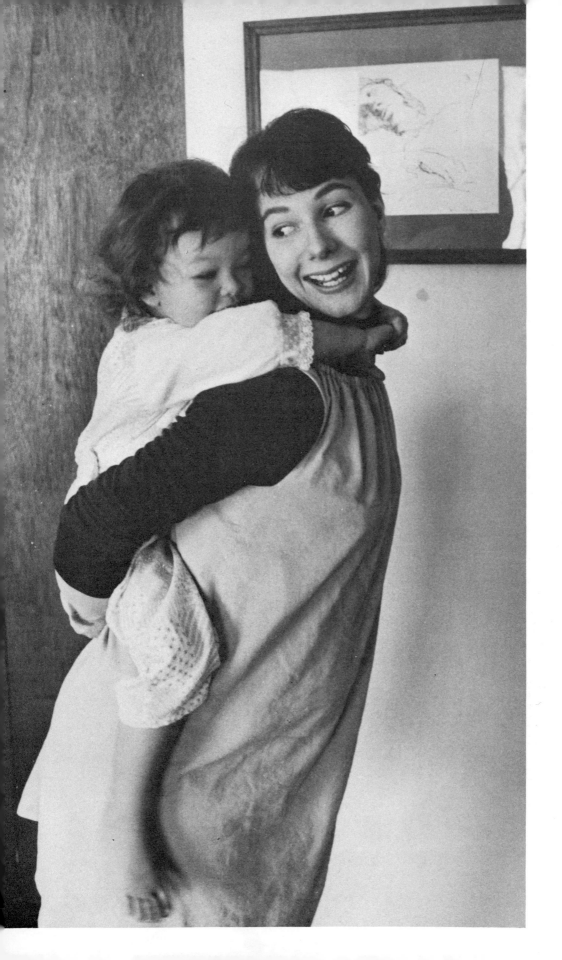

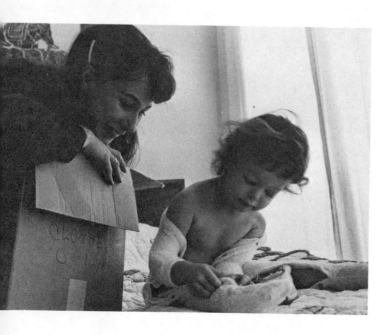

Kim's baby clothers had been carefully stored. As they are brought out, Kim rediscovers a forgotten favorite. Now big enough to fasten the snaps, she is much too big to wear the tiny pajamas. Realizing this, Kim suggested they would be just right for the new baby. She asked if a boy baby or a girl baby could wear the same clothes.

Following the group discussion at a monthly La Leche League meeting, Cathy Talcott visits with Charlotte. Kim has long-since gone to sleep on the couch.

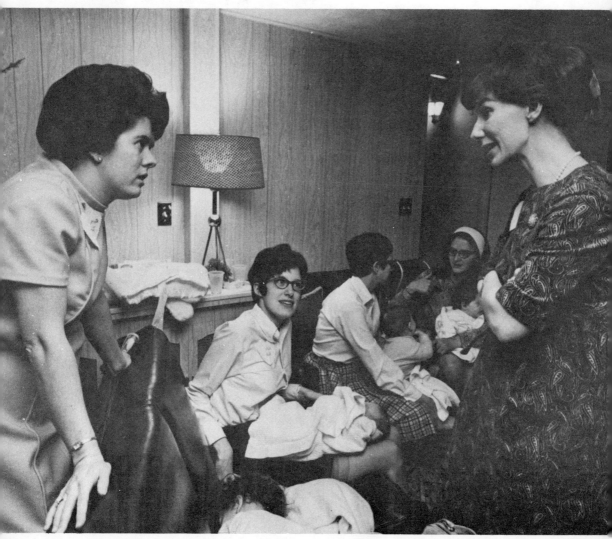

Just as childbirth is not an end in itself, neither is it a beginning. It is at once a going and a coming. Having a joyful experience prepares the mother for an instinctive response to nurture her infant. Breastfeeding is the continuation of an urgent symbiosis between child and mother, between child and father, and ultimately between child and family.

According to nature's logic, the baby needs food and the mother needs to give. The baby needs warmth, assurance, gentleness; both mother and father have strong and willing arms to provide for these needs. The infant is cradled in the lap of tradition, and grows to wonder about his world and his place in this world; his family's unique wisdom and love provide him with his education and his faith by example and counsel. And, as Arthur Koestler has written, "a Faith is not acquired by reasoning; . . . it grows like a tree. Its crown points to the sky; its roots grow downward into the past and are nourished by the dark sap of the ancestral humus."

With warmth I still remember summering on my grandmother's homestead when I was a child. There I saw the farm hands carry their babies with them into the fields and settle them to nap in pasteboard boxes under the shade trees. I watched the mothers respond to their own children's need and nurse the babies while they themselves rested in the cool. Once I heard the older women in my family talk about Gladys Johnson having a "good farm birth" and how her husband, Roby, had been by her side to help out. At the time, it was inconceivable to me that such impressions would have relevance to me later in adult life. Now I realize that the information I received then, and countless other images I can no longer recall consciously made a deep impression on me. And the sum of all my past experiences will in turn be available to my children and my children's children. I find it intensely exciting to be an integral link between my past and my future family.

Distilled to the essence, I want to take responsibility for myself as the childbearer so that I can protect the coming baby. I want to claim the human traditions of birth, not the institutional interferences, and I want to share these traditions in a personal and creative experience with my family.

So it is that I look back to the time eight-and-a-half years ago when I was first pregnant. I am glad for what wisdom I did have, sorry for what wisdom I didn't. As a young wife in a "nuclear" family, I missed out on day-to-day contact with much of the guidance traditionally handed down through the family. My husband Fred and I discussed childbirth with contemporaries and read books, mostly in the field of child care. Unfortunately, I chose an obstetrician for his proximity, not his philosophy. He suggested a hospital where he was on the staff. Although I approached my first labor full of anticipation, I lacked critical details. Despite intuitive reservations, I accepted what came. Fred was asked to leave the labor room and I didn't see him again until after the baby was born. Natural childbirth was alien to the doctor and the nurses who attended me. The baby was taken away from me immediately after birth and put in a nursery for the first seven hours of her life. Rooming-in was not permitted; feedings were on an enforced four-hour schedule; breastfeeding was treated without special considerations or supports.

Perhaps some ancient maternal ancestor brandished a tribal amulet to protect the baby and me. At any rate, large measures of my body's own oxytocin and prolactin (hormones) in combination with the thoughts of Grantly Dick-Read and

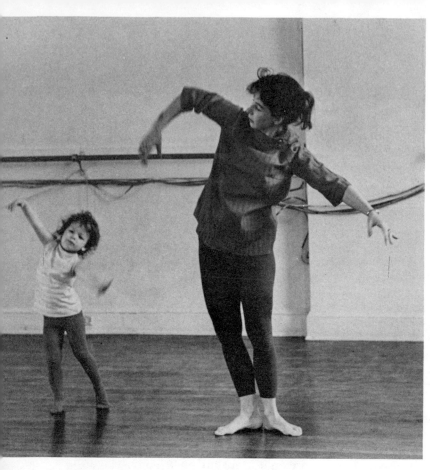

Feeling that exercise and activity would contribute to good health and an easy birth, Charlotte continued modern dance class throughout her pregnancy. Kim looked forward to her occasional visits to the studio with her mother.

After Dr. Brew has finished examining Charlotte, Kim wants a turn on the table. Playing "doctor" fascinated her and helped her learn what to expect.

Margaret Ribble, an analyst in NYC, (pioneers in the area of natural childbirth) carried us through the hospital delivery relatively unscathed. Still, every interference has its price, and I will never be quite sure what might have been had I been allowed to proceed at my own pace. I had a good, firm labor—in spite of the hormone ordered by the doctor to speed my contractions, in spite of his rupturing my membranes during the second hour of labor, in spite of the episiotomy. Neither the need for or the consequences of these "routine" procedures was explained. Pain killers were offered, but I turned them down. Without drugs, my first daughter Kim appeared alert and wonderfully healthy. She and I managed to learn breastfeeding on the hospital schedule.

On the second night in the hospital, I awoke at 2:30 A.M. with a start and realized that Kim had not been brought to me for her feeding. When I rang and

asked for her, the nurse explained that I had been asleep at 2:00 and that it was now too late. She didn't want to get the baby "off schedule." I found it incomprehensible that my day-and-a-half-old baby even *had* a schedule in the first place! I found it inhumane that I was reduced to tears and threats before the nurse finally relented and brought Kim to me.

Two days later, a blizzard notwithstanding, Fred and I assembled our family and went home. His mother, who stayed to help us for several weeks, shared with us her reservoir of information. Fred had been born at home and she had nursed him, so she had much to give.

I also joined La Leche League for help in nursing Kim. In one of the monthly meetings, a Childbirth Education Association (C.E.A.) member told the story of her recent home delivery. Discovering a home birth was still possible, I could

11

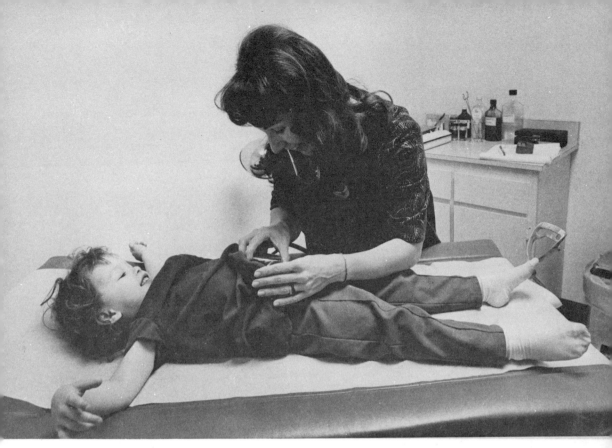

hardly wait to tell Fred the news. Over the months, the more we read and thought about the possibility, the more convinced we became that our next child had to be born at home. Not only did I look forward to having Fred and Kim present but also I was very sensitive to the advantages of undisturbed and unrestricted interaction between the mother and the new baby.

Word travels fast of any doctor who practices the natural methods so dear to the hearts of many League women. In this way I learned about an obstetrician, Dr. James Brew, on the C.E.A. board, a friend of the League, the only doctor in town who did a selected few home deliveries each year. After I became pregnant Fred and I went to see Dr. Brew. He assured us that if I remained in excellent health and that if we did not change our minds, we could plan on a home birth.

Since Kim's untrained, unmedicated

birth had been such a positive experience, I decided not to enroll in childbirth classes but to go on taking modern dance lessons, usually two or three a week. The teacher and other students accepted me. Sometimes they kidded me, occasionally fussed over me when they thought I was exceeding my more and more limited range. Kim went with me when there was no baby sitter available and tried to do the barre work and dance routines.

Fred and I read many books over the nine months, this time concentrating on prepared childbirth, exercises and breathing techniques, and some history and philosophy of childbirth. We included Kim in our discussions, and she went with me to see Dr. Brew. After watching the examinations carefully, she wanted to lie down on the table and play patient with me. I would examine her little stomach and listen with the stethoscope and pronounce her condition "extraordinary!" Then we would meet with Dr.

12

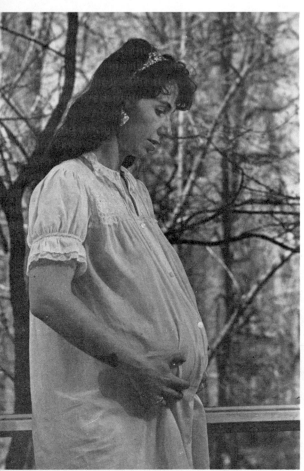

Brew in his office. He always took time to be attentive to Kim and gave me all the time I asked for, listening, answering questions, and making plans. Back at home, Kim and her friends could be overheard playing doctor with Kim repeating Dr. Brew's instructions verbatim.

We were eager for the time to arrive. Just after midnight on a soft April evening, I awakened to the gentle tugging of contractions. Lying still, I felt them sweep over me for an hour before waking

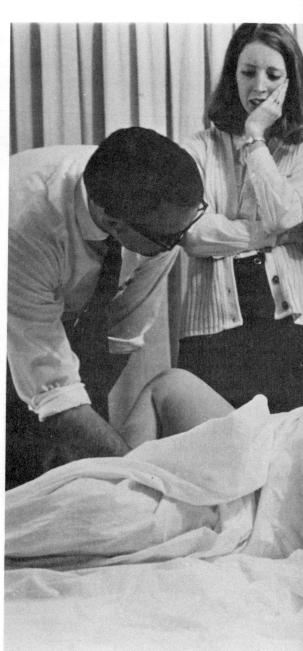

Nearing the end of the first stage of labor, Charlotte (above) still prefers walking as the most comfortable position. She practices effluerage and controlled breathing during a contraction. Soon after, Dr. Brew (right) determines that dilatation is almost complete and transition near. Mikie Donohue, nurse assistant, sympathizes about a burning sensation.

Fred. I got dressed, and even put on makeup for the camera. Fred is a professional photographer and we didn't intend to miss the opportunity to capture on film an event as important as the birth of our baby. While I called Mikie Donohue, the C.E.A. nurse who was to assist Dr. Brew, and a friend, Ritva Hackel, Fred organized the room for pictures. Days before he had put up strobes and placed cameras on tripods, an amusing sight to friends who had seen the equipment in

place in our bedroom. We then prepared refreshments for the morning ahead—sandwiches and whole wheat banana bread, fresh-squeezed orange juice and coffee.

Mikie arrived about 2:30 A.M. and Ritva about 3:00. After Mikie determined that I was five centimeters dilated, she called the doctor, who sleepily appeared on the scene at 3:30. His examination suggested I was progressing slowly, so he promptly asked for a bed so that he

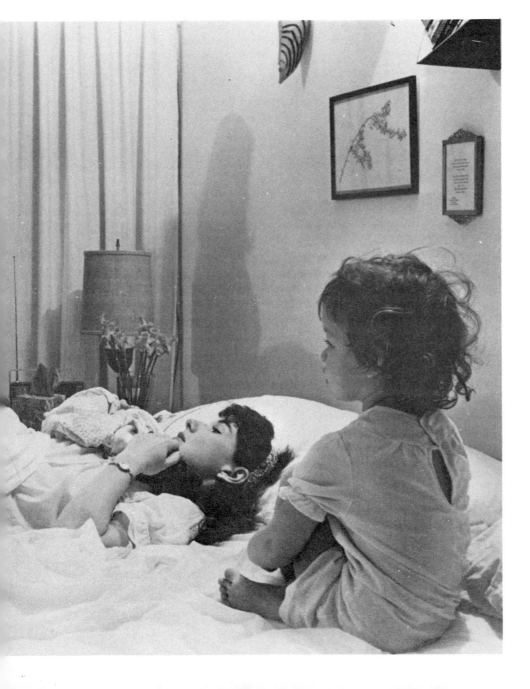

could get some more sleep before the birth. By this time Kim had awakened in the flurry of activity; she generously offered her bed to Dr. Brew. He slept there until morning, then left for his hospital rounds and office appointments.

In the meantime, there we all sat with little to do. Kim, our dog Boo and her pup, Poopsie, all curled up on the bed beside me for long naps. Breaking to take an occasional picture, Fred and I passed the time pleasantly until dawn. With Mikie and Ritva, the mood of the night was much like a slumber party when I was a young girl—we were all tired but too excited to sleep. Every hour or so Mikie would do an examination, always discouragingly similar to the one before. I had anticipated a quick and easy labor, but time passed and my cervix opened very slowly.

During the night my contractions built in intensity and were painful at times. This came as a complete surprise to me, since Kim's birth had been so free from discomfort that I had gained an enormous self-confidence. Mikie and Fred put powder on their hands and took turns applying a firm rubbing pressure to the small of my back. Though a great relief to me, this must have been tiring for them. Standing up was most comfortable, but a hard position for me to maintain overnight. I was miserable lying down, so I spent most of the time walking about, going upstairs to eat, or sitting on the bed Indian-style. To keep up my energy I consumed glassfuls of orange juice mixed with high-protein powder and bowlfuls of yogurt.

Kim stayed close by me most of the morning, occasionally taking time out to chat with visitors in the kitchen, nibble at the refreshments, and let the dogs in and out of the door. The rest of the time she played with her toys next to me. When she began jumping and bouncing

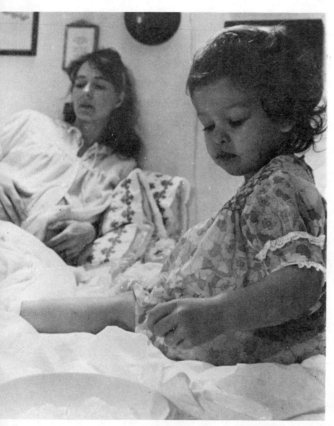

Kim is ready with ice chips as her mother breathes through the discomfort of a transition stage contraction.

on the bed, Fred produced a bag of "treasures" we had thought to collect earlier in the week. Other diversions came in an Easter package from her grandparents—small toys and a fancy dress.

I grew hot and thirsty as the morning dragged on. Kim wanted a job and proved very helpful in cooling my washcloth and handing me ice chips. Although I needed quiet during contractions, her kisses and hugs and general thoughtfulness more than made up for the jiggles and jogs. The Lamaze breathing techniques were useful, and Mikie coached me when I faltered. I was glad I had read and danced so much but regretted my decision not to take the C.E.A. instruction. But never did I regret not being in the hospital. I was glad to be with Fred and Kim and have the friendly, warm feeling that goes with being "at home."

By 11 A.M. the contractions were very strong. I was nearing transition when Mikie called Dr. Brew back to the house. Everyone looked tired and a bit blurry, but we rallied when he appeared. I suppose we realized that we wouldn't have long to wait now.

With little advance notice, the transition stage of labor began. Responding to the first deep, guttural groan of the pushing stage, I automatically began to bear down. Everyone rushed in to help me, and just in time for on the third such contraction, I felt as if I would break open, actually burst apart. I demanded of Dr. Brew, "Tell me what to do! What should I *do*?" He responded firmly, "Pant—push—push very gently—a quarter is showing!"

Somewhere beyond the din inside of me, I heard Kim wail. It was hard to focus on her, but I finally realized that she wanted to climb on the bed beside me and that her way was blocked by Dr. Brew's table of instruments. Then Fred came to her rescue. I knew he was taking pictures and hugging Kim at the same time. "Now it's a half dollar—PANT!" "Oh, God!" I heard myself cry. "Push gently—the head is coming—it's born, the head is out!" "It's BORN! Oh, Fred, our baby is *BORN*!" I clutched Ritva's hand, called out to Fred, though I knew he couldn't come and leave Kim and the cameras untended. He cried out and through the chaos of my senses his voice came, "The shoulder is out—PUSH!" and with one enormous effort, like the eruption of a volcano, the baby burst forth.

Instantly I felt utter relief and fantastic emptiness. The baby was before me, head down, and crying. I was exhausted but alive, very alive and aware. And in a voice I will never forget, Fred exclaimed to me, "It's a *boy*, Charley!" We held hands and Kim clambered across the bed to snuggle beside my head. I gave her a kiss and a tight hug, assuring her that everything was just fine.

Holding the baby close for me to see, Dr. Brew milked the cord and clamped it. Then he gently explained that the postnatal examination would take only a few minutes. Wistfully I looked toward the table, anxious to make contact with the baby again. Momentarily the little one was handed down to me, bright and pink with a full and hardy appearance. When he stretched he looked like Fred. My love enveloped him as he snuggled against me. Homing in by instinct, he rooted for my nipple and diligently began to nurse. I was used to Kim's mouth, strong from three years of practice. There seemed to be confidence in the grasp of this small tight mouth, and his trust was expressed by a sigh. Apparently content with his welcome, he fell asleep.

Our catharsis was an exulted recounting of our feelings. Fred and Kim and I celebrated together. We settled on the

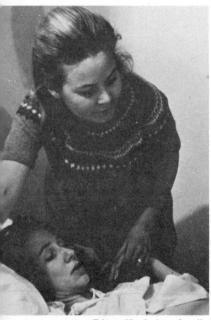

Ritva Hackel, a family friend and nurse, offers support as the baby is born. This kind of warmth and additional assistance was a considerable contrast to Charlotte's hospital delivery of Kim. This is one of the main reasons she prefers home birth.

Birth—the long awaited moment! A final push brought forth a boy—Christopher. Having grown more interested as the activity increased, Kim moved around to the end of the bed. Mikie answers her question as she bends low for a look at the baby's face.

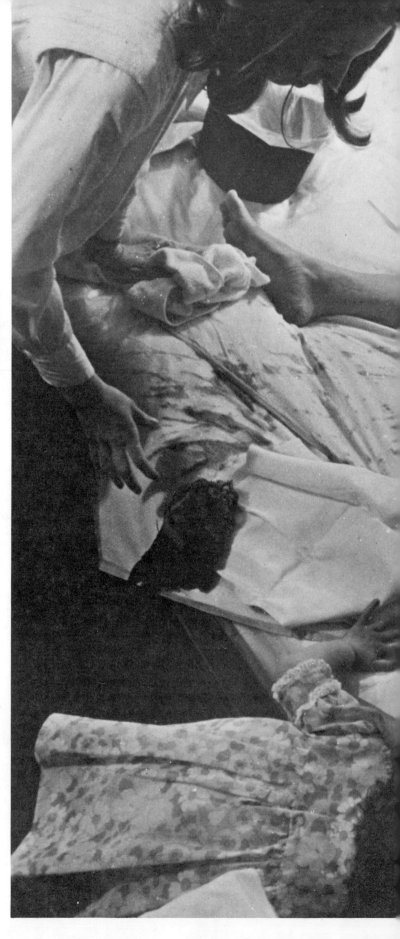

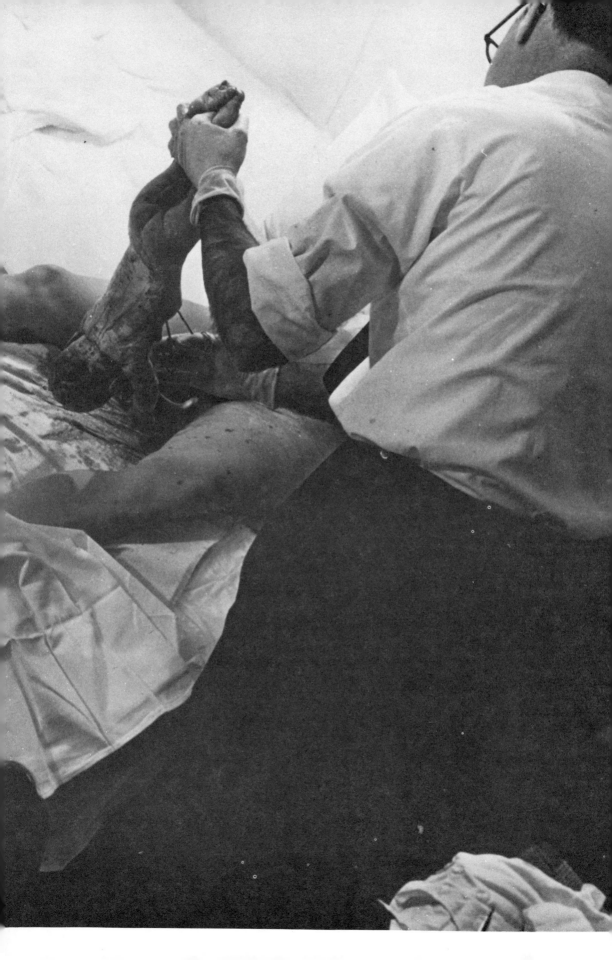

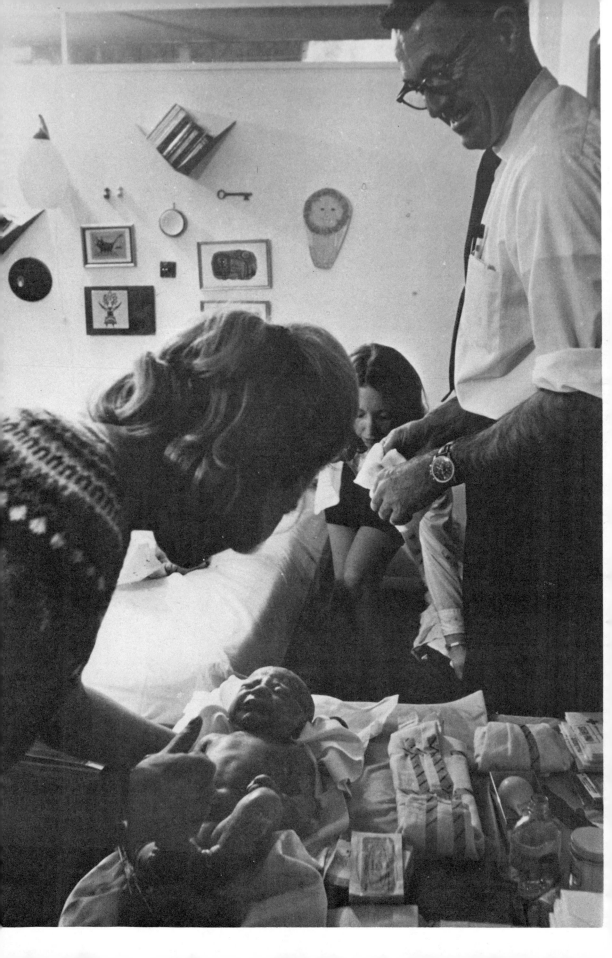

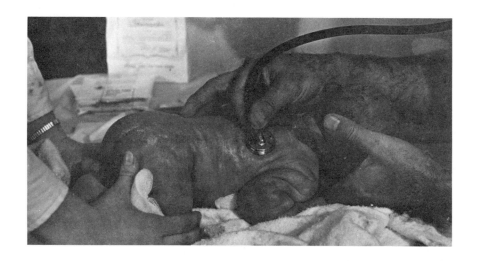

Ritva gently settles newborn Christopher for an initial examination. Then moments later, Mikie hands him down to Charlotte. Holding the baby for the first time evokes a singular joy. This immediate closeness allows mother and child and other members of the family to establish a bond of life and love with the new baby.

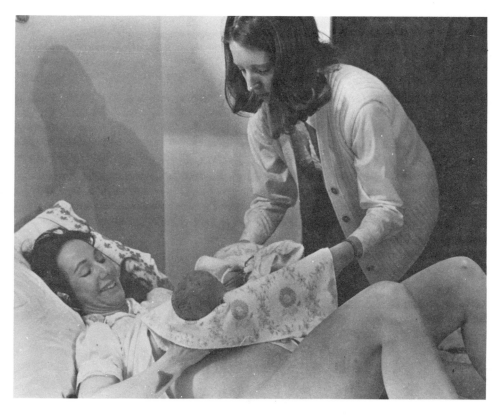

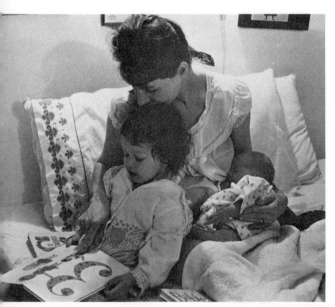

Content with nursing, Christopher sleeps. An hour after the birth and a refreshing shower, Charlotte is able to devote special time to Kim.

first name *Christopher,* Kim's choice, and *David,* after Fred's paternal grandfather. I requested a peanut butter and apple butter sandwich and a glass of milk. Then, as everyone else snacked in the kitchen, I showered and changed clothes. Our friends were all gone by three o'clock. We called our families, I nursed Christopher from time to time, and Fred cooked a delicious dinner of liver and eggs for three tired people. Bedtime at 7:00 found us exhausted and very content.

Ashley Montagu once punned that for the first nine months after birth, a child should be provided "a womb with a view," and this is exactly what I tried to give Christopher. He was nursed on request and taken with me wherever I went. As he grew, people sometimes stopped to ask me about the baby carrier I used and fretted about my comfort. I retold this story: A youngster at Boys Town, U.S.A. was carrying another child almost as large as he. But when the director came upon them and expressed concern for his load, the young boy answered clearly, "He's not heavy, Father, he's my brother." My mothering Christopher made us both happy.

What we have done is not really extraordinary in the history of man, but it is unusual in our civilized society. How ironic that trying to perpetuate the race by nature's laws runs counter to what over 95 percent of the American people accept as right and proper. So we run the risk of eccentricity in trying to find our way safely between what many now decry as "out-moded nonsense," on the one hand, and what we object to as "medical over-reaction," on the other.

Home birth for me is neither an act of bravery nor of foolhardiness. It is a seriously considered choice—*my* choice for bearing my babies in dignity and self-respect so that I can remember my birth experiences with joy and, gaining sustenance from them, mother the children of my womb. For me, home birth is a commitment of love.

21

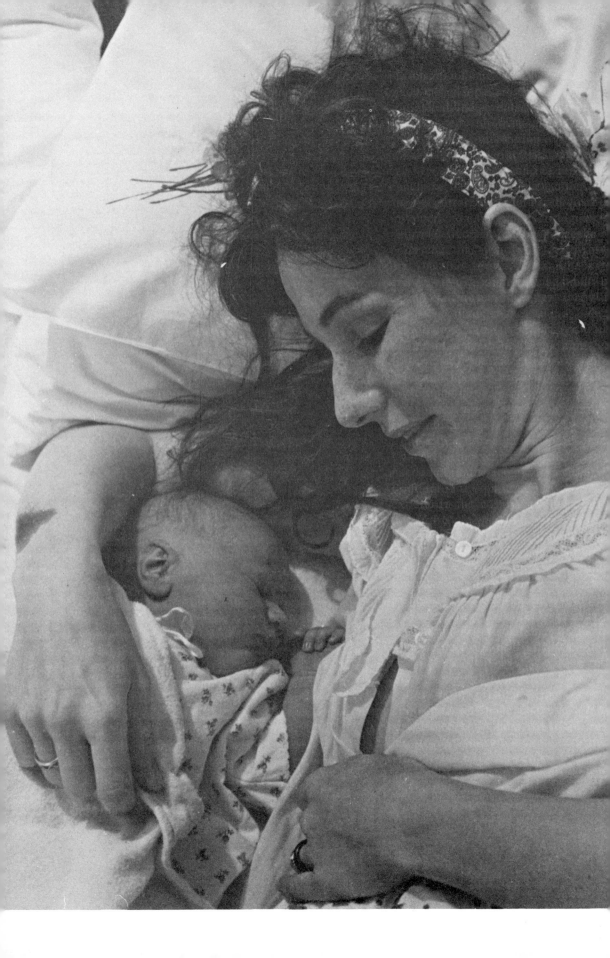

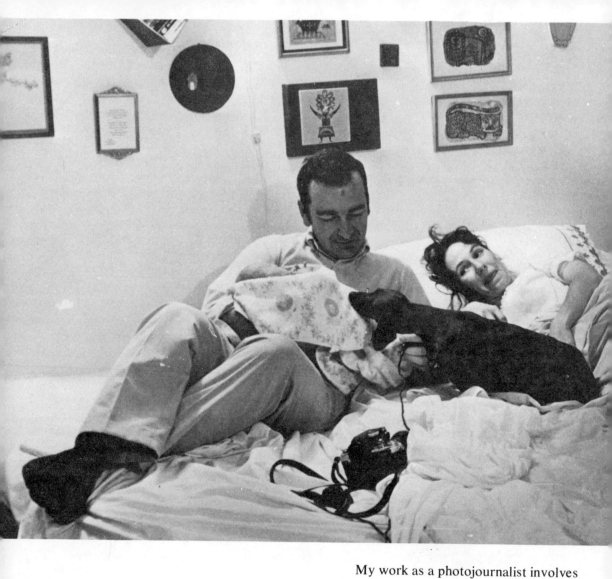

Fred's Story

BY FRED WARD

My work as a photojournalist involves travel throughout the world. I have always considered these experiences in other lands as the broadest and the best educational tools possible. Since I became interested in births and families about ten years ago, I started looking seriously into the customs of the countries I visited. One of the basic findings was that, with few exceptions, families were brought together by a birth. Mothers and fathers were physically near and certainly seemed to be emotionally involved in a way that made me question the accepted mid-century traditions of childbirth.

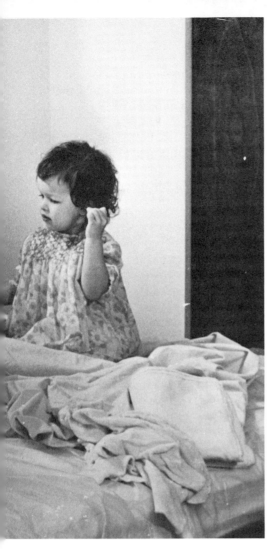

Fred lays down his cameras to hold his son, while Boo, the family pet, checks out the new baby. This is a peaceful time for everyone following the excitment of a twelve-hour labor and birth. Now there is time to savor the good experience.

On trying to analyze family customs and mores in the United States, I realized that the current condition is relatively new. Historically, our country developed along the lines of immigrant cultures that melted into it. For over a century, frontier determination, extended families, home births, breastfeeding, and numerous children were all facets of American life. Then changes began to take place in that structure. As the leader of the world's industrialization, America also led the way toward a new kind of family. Children moved away to form smaller "nuclear" family units. Old folks were put into separate homes instead of living out their lives among their children and grandchildren with whom they, and they alone, could share their specific wisdom and sense of continuity. It became unpopular to have more than two children, and, all too often, breastfeeding was looked down on as being low-class and not the "modern" thing to do. Home births became only a fading memory from the 1920s and '30s except for some big city ghetto residents and the Southern mountaineers.

It was during my period of historical examination that several events combined to bring a new view into sharp focus. My wife and I had become interested in natural foods about the time that Charlotte became pregnant with our first baby, Kim. I was impressed with the literature on the benefits of organic foods because it seemed logical to me and it also fit into what I considered to be my "natural approach" to life. With that in mind, I was not surprised at all to find that Charlotte began talking about a "natural" delivery. An unmedicated birth seemed highly desirable, and the decision to breastfeed was a reasonable continuation of our concern for nutrition for our baby.

It was the medical aspect of this first pregnancy that ultimately fixed our ideas for the future. This was 1966, and even though I had been born at home, we knew no contemporaries who were.

24

Certainly we did not know of any doctors in the Washington area who were delivering outside hospitals. As many young couples do we followed the recommendation of a friend and contacted a nearby obstetrician. He turned out to be "traditional and conservative," meaning quite paradoxically that he rejected all but the last few decades of our country's birth customs. Offering no support or information, he reluctantly agreed to let Charlotte have her way with an unmedicated birth.

For nine months I watched Charlotte grow from the wife I had loved for years into a first-time mother. It was a remarkable development that permeated her whole being and personality. I, too, felt myself changing. I had new concerns for more time and space, anxiety over increased responsibilities a family would bring, fears about Charlotte and my loss of privacy and mobility. But nature has incredible force, working in unique and unfathomable paths to cope with constantly evolving circumstances. I found that as Charlotte visibly became a mother, I was feeling and thinking more like a father. We had shared in the conception and were now sharing in the initial growth. The climax was still to come and promised to be the best experience of all.

And yet—somehow—the culture of the 1960s got in the way. The sharing of the greatest single experience in the lives of a couple was about to be denied because somehow, somewhere, other people had decided that it was not valid anymore. "Didn't anyone ever tell you, husbands are not allowed to be with their wives at birth. Hospitals cannot allow that. Besides, obstetricians would not put up with that. Why would you want to see that anyway? Do it the way they do it in the movies. Pace outside and smoke a lot." Incredible!

Youth and inexperience were unfortunate companions in our case. We did not know any better and could find no support for an alternative. So we reluctantly went to the hospital. After I filled out the interminable forms and paid a sizeable deposit, I delivered Charlotte to the labor room door. That was the last I saw of her as a young, pregnant woman. Except for her no one cared whether I was there or not. In fact, I got the distinct impression from the staff that they wished I would leave. I remember thinking that a taxi driver depositing a woman in labor probably pleased the hospital staff most of all. That would be most efficient and impersonal.

As ridiculous as the formalities were, they were only the prelude to endless other insensitive procedures and practices. Although our experience was in no way as frightening as others we have heard about, it was enough to alter our lives. I will never forget standing in stark disbelief at not being allowed to be in the same room as our new daughter. I had to look through the protective glass into the nursery, a room filled with pathetic, crying infants being systematically fed with water or formula in bottles. I stood wondering why those babies could not be held and nursed by their mothers with their fathers present; I left close to tears. By this time, I had read enough to know that any germs the new babies might get would almost surely come from their being born in a hospital and not from their mothers or fathers.

I was angered beyond words when Charlotte related her continuing struggles with the nurses who resisted her desire to have our child in her room so that the baby could be held, snuggled, and nursed. I wanted out of the hospital, and I wanted our baby out, and I never wanted to go back. There are no ways adequate to express the helpless, frustrating feelings I had when I encountered such perplexing logic—where it seemed the hospital rules denied my rights as a father, to say nothing of my child's birthright. No one who has ever observed a mother animal fiercely protecting her young could question the motives of a concerned new mother fighting the hospital system to have her baby with her.

Like millions of other fathers I felt cheated. What right did anyone have to exclude me? I drove my wife to the hospital and returned four days later to drive home a family. The time between was ripped from my family's storehouse of shared experiences. We were not allowed to be together for one of the most intimate moments in our lives.

This trauma made us decide that something was seriously wrong in our culture as it related to birth and that we did not want to participate in this wrenching and "unnatural" act again. On the positive side, it coalesced our resolve to find a way to have a home birth. Before the advent of the second pregnancy three years later, our search had been rewarded. We found Dr. Brew, who accepted a limited number of home births, and he agreed to our request. The whole tone of the pregnancy was affected. We felt relieved, relaxed, and casual.

Besides the enormous advantage of being able to share the birth experience in our own way, the major improvement over the first delivery would be my increased awareness of the birth process and an involvement in husband-coached labor. Since a home birth is unmedicated, the woman should prepare herself to work with the sensations of labor. Her husband keeps track of the contractions, notes the duration, and calls the level of breathing. Not incidental is the psychological support that passes between husband and wife. This team effort is marvelously successful in keeping the couple closely involved in their joint project.

Fred takes special time with Kim at the library in order to keep her feeling important as an individual and involved.

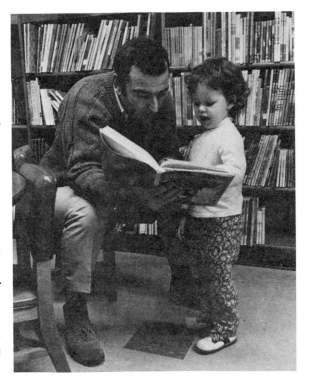

We made another decision as the delivery drew near. I am a photographer by profession. We talked about photographs and agreed that it would be a loss to our family if I passed up the opportunity to document our home birth. Naturally I felt it would be a challenge and a wonderful experience, but it would take me away from participating fully as a labor coach. Charlotte and I concluded that her own independence, reading, and experience gave her sufficient confidence to carry on without my actually coaching the birth. We also were assured that Dr. Brew and Mickie Donohue, the nurse who would assist him, would take over that function. I planned to photograph all during labor, delivery, and into the first days of our new baby's life.

I stopped taking out-of-town assignments three weeks before the estimated birth-day. When the time seemed near, I prepared the bedroom for photography. Electronic flash units were installed to be permanent and unobtrusive. Two electrically operated remote cameras covered the room from angles where I could not be. Everything checked out, and I felt my part was ready.

I cannot overstate my admiration for Charlotte's will, resolve, strength, and tenderness during the day of Chris' birth. This was her "special time" and nothing could detract from it. She was up walking around, wanting to take care of Kim and me and, ultimately, our medical friends. I would not say I felt completely useless, but she was so well organized and self-reliant that there was practically nothing for me to do directly relating to the impending birth. Except for bringing yogurt, and later ice, and talking quietly with her, I busied myself wholly with photographing the events. At several rough periods, Charlotte wanted to hold hands and be close to me. I gave my loving support. But mainly she knew what

she was doing and proceeded straight away to her project—having a baby.

Over the years I have often thought about those moments of closeness. When a man sees his woman working as hard as she does during labor and watches stress crease her forehead, he has an irresistible urge to support her. Repeatedly I thought back to Kim's hospital birth and regretted I had not been there beside Charlotte when she needed me. Once the contractions started coming close together I never left the bedroom, and I constantly sensed that each of us appreciated the warm comfort of just knowing that the other was so near.

I have relived those exhilarating seconds a thousand times. As I look back over the many photographs, I can still recall my surprise and excitement when our newborn baby Chris practically flew into Dr. Brew's waiting hands. Chris lay shiny and dripping with his warm protective coating still covering his unfolded little body. Even before his first cry notifying the world that he was born, I could not hold back my joy and said, "Oh, Charley, it's a boy!"

Three years later when our third child was born, there was never any doubt: the only answer was birth at home. Now our family is complete. If we ever do have other children we will continue to seek this same kind of family sharing. Our home births have been among the most rewarding experiences in our married lives. I have never tried to convince others to follow our way. When people ask, I try to tell them our story and what it has meant to me—two memorable events of great happiness and remarkable beauty.

Christopher's thirty-minute-old feet— still wrinkled from being wet. The tiny toes seem to define their new space by constant wriggling and flexing.

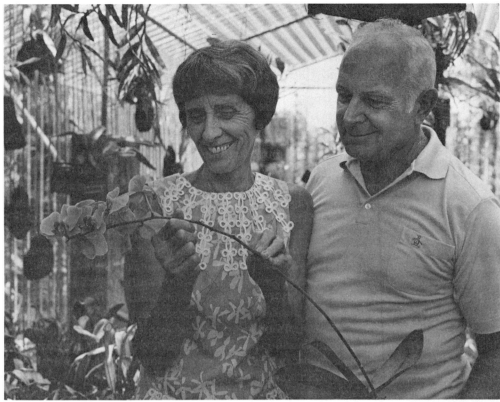

PHOTO BY RAY FISHER

Fred's parents, Bess and Newman Ward. Fred, who was born at home in Huntsville, Alabama, questions his parents on their home birth experience in this interview. Mr. Ward has recently retired from the U.S. Postal Service; Mrs. Ward is active in garden clubs and conservation groups. Their hobby is raising orchids.

BESS: Dr. Jordon explained what the birth would be like, and I read some books. He told me to eat well so I'd have a good pregnancy and plenty of milk. My mother was an organic gardener like you all, Fred. We had a cow and chickens, so they fertilized the garden. I ate a lot of fresh vegetables and fruit, and I loved buttermilk.

NEWMAN: She had the prettiest complexion you ever saw.

FRED: Had you ever seen a birth?

BESS: No, I never had, but I've been around babies all my life. Mama had all five of us at home. Daddy always took us children to my aunt's house when the baby was being born, but that was just for the day. When I was 11, Juanita was born. I remember bathing her and taking her back to the bed to Mama. They kept a woman in bed for two weeks then. I grew up taking care of babies and washing "dad-gummed" diapers.

NEWMAN: Bess was the oldest and she helped take care of all the others.

BESS: There was one thing that worried me about your birth.

FRED: Oh, really? What's that?

BESS: Well, on the Saturday before you were born on Tuesday, I was sitting in the porch swing when Dub came running up to tell me something. He flopped down beside me. He was a great big old boy, you know, he was in high school at the time. The swing broke and we hit the floor! It just scared Mama to death. She thought sure it had injured the baby. It didn't seem to bother you, but you were born soon after that.

FRED: Was I due?

BESS: No, you were about five weeks early.

FRED: That might have had something to do with it then.

BESS: Mama always said it did.

FRED: How much did I weigh?

BESS: You weighed eight pounds. About the first month of your life, you slept about all the time. I'd have to wake you up to feed you. I'd get too full with milk and start hurting, so I'd wake you up to nurse.

FRED: Tell me about the birth.

BESS: Your daddy and I were playing gin rummy that night with Dub and Brooks.

FRED: Dub and Brooks lived there, too?

BESS: Yes, Dub was still in high school and Brooks wasn't married yet. We kept running outside to watch the eclipse. There was an eclipse of the moon that night. Then we'd go in and play another hand and run back out again. After the moon was out full, everybody went to bed. It must have been past midnight.

I woke up about 3 A.M. with the pains. I figured something was happening, so Newman woke Mama.

NEWMAN: Then I walked to the nurse's station where there was a telephone and asked the nurse to call Dr. Jordon. The pains were about 15 to 20 minutes apart, and we figured he should come soon. We watched for him the whole time, expected him any minute. About six o'clock I went back to the nursing home again and told the nurse the pains were closer—about 10 minutes apart then. She called him while I was there. In fact, I waited to make sure. I heard her speak to him. Dr. Jordon got to the house in about 20 minutes. Bess was ready when he got there.

FRED: How long was he there before I was born?

BESS: I guess about 20 minutes. Yes, it seems to me that's what Mama said. She told him she was scared because he'd gotten there so close to the birth.

Anyway, everything went smoothly. Mama was on one side of the bed and your daddy was on the other. I remember I had a lot of pillows all propped up under my head.

NEWMAN: The doctor told us to get on each side and for her to pull on us when she was trying to force out the baby. We held hands the whole time.

FRED: Did he give you any drugs?

BESS: Just a little choloroform, nothing else. He put a mask over my nose, and I tried to push it away. It made me feel like I was choking.

NEWMAN: I got so sleepy that I could hardly sit up.

31

BESS: I think Dr. Jordon saw he was putting Newman out, so he just put the mask aside. I never lost consciousness. I was helping myself all the time. And when he held you up and I saw you, I didn't think about myself at all. I just saw you and wanted to make sure you were all right.

NEWMAN: The doctor held you upside down and you cried.

BESS: I was leery about that. I was afraid the doctor would drop you, holding you with both feet in one hand like that, but he didn't. You gave just a short little cry. When he was cutting the cord, I remember telling him to be careful. I didn't want him to hurt you. Mama asked if you needed to be circumcised. He said, "No. I don't do it unless there's something wrong." I never could bring myself to have it done. Then he put some drops into your eyes. I was watching every move. I was going to make sure he didn't do anything to you.

Mama rolled you up in a towel and took you downstairs to bathe you. She already had everything laid out on the kitchen table. I heard you crying and that worried me. I asked Newman to see if everything was all right. I was very concerned. Then she brought you back upstairs in a little white nightgown. I can still see the way you looked. She put you in bed with me. You had your eyes open and looked up at me. I wanted to hold you. I remember holding you, and I said, "Look at the curls!" You had them right on the top of your head. They were wet where Mama had washed you. We looked at you feet. They were so tiny.

FRED: Did you nurse me on a schedule?

BESS: No, Honey, I didn't. I just let you eat when you wanted to. I had a little bassinet for you. We sold it when we came to Miami. We used it for you and then for Lynn, after she was born. I'd pull it right up beside the bed. I guess the first year of your life, I slept with my hand in it all night so that if you moved, I could feel you.

FRED: How long did I nurse?

BESS: Until you were about 15 months old.

FRED: How do you remember the birth process?

BESS: They told me it was an easy birth. I didn't need any stitches. I can't remember all of the conversation, but Dr. Jordon did say, "It went smoothly."

They made you stay in bed for two weeks in those days, except I'd get up and sit in a chair if there was no one else in the room, or sit on the side of the bed. You know me, Fred, I don't like to stay in bed. Besides, I wasn't even sore after you were born.

FRED: I'd like to hear what happened that day, the day I was born.

NEWMAN: I stayed at home about an hour after you were born. Then I walked over to tell Mom and Pop the news. They lived about a mile away, so I stopped by on the way to work. I told all of the boys down at the Y about you. I said, "It's a boy." I was so proud. I was wishing for a boy.

BESS: It really didn't matter to me. Just so it was all right, I didn't care.

NEWMAN: We were happy because everything went so perfectly. You were perfect, and the delivery went well.

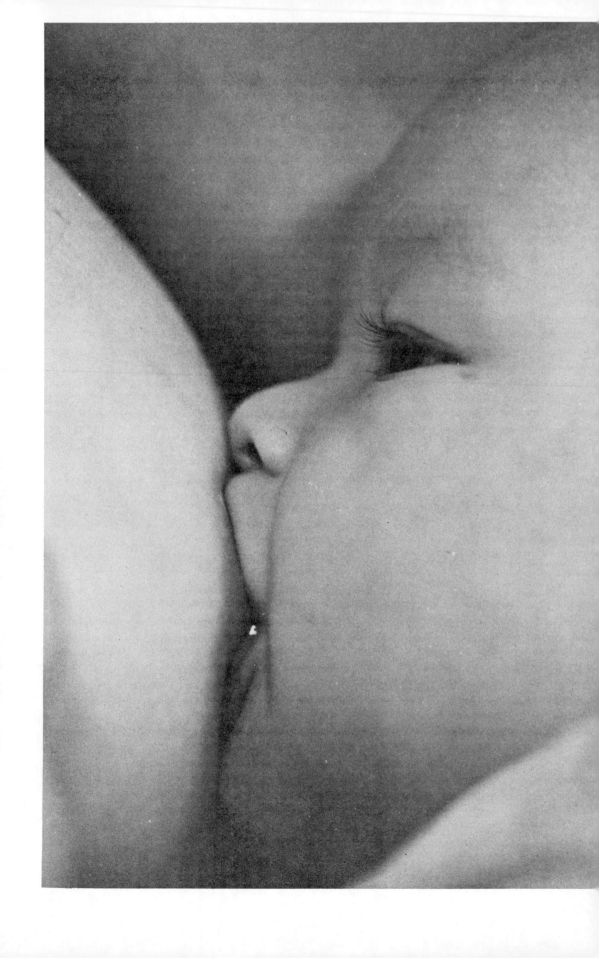

part 2

The Medical and Psychological Dimension

By James D. Brew, M.D.

An Öbstetrician's Point of View

For over two decades I delivered babies in the homes of families in and around Washington, D.C., where I practice obstetrics and gynecology. When I delivered my first baby at home in the mid-1950s, it was because a patient had asked me to do so, not because I was crusading to change the accepted birth practices in this country where well over 95 percent of all births are in hospitals. I had come to believe strongly that families should have a choice of birth styles and that they should make the key decision as to where they wanted their child born and as to whether they wished a medicated hospital delivery or an unmedicated natural childbirth.

Birth is a family affair, and the doctor should assist a family in this milestone event rather than dictate the terms of the occasion. Some families want unmedicated or natural deliveries in a hospital setting with the father present; others want natural childbirth in the home setting. I believe in supplying what my patients ask for, provided, of course, there are no medical complications. Over a time, I foresee that more families will consider the home as a safe alternative to the hospital for the birth of their children. I have found that home delivery is a rewarding experience for me, but more importantly, that it has proved enriching for the families involved.

Background

My medical practice—obstetrics and gynecology (OB-GYN)—began in Washington in 1953. Requests for home delivery came mainly from some of my Christian Science patients. Because of their beliefs, they wanted to avoid organized medicine as much as possible; but they still wanted competent medical help available. After some research and reflection, I agreed to their requests. In 1956, I delivered six babies at home. Word spread and many of my patients who were not Christian Scientists started asking for home deliveries. Wherever possible I worked them into my schedule. This was new to me and there was very little information or help to use as a guide. So, I thought the best thing to do would be to proceed slowly. Each year I would limit the home births to under a dozen. I got more requests than that, but I was training help and doing all the patient training and that was about all I could handle.

Following the initial demand by my Christian Science patients, the year in and year out requests for home delivery came from couples who were trained or at least interested in the various natural childbirth methods. This is only to be expected since in a home situation we prefer to have a non-medicated delivery. I was also very active in organizations that favored natural childbirth and breast-feeding, and people in these groups often learned through the grapevine of some other family who had lived through a home birth experience. Before groups like the Childbirth Education Association became established, however, I taught my own childbirth preparation classes.

I did this for my patients and to help me understand the processes and benefits of natural deliveries. One thing I wanted to find was why I was getting so much more involved with these home deliveries than I was with the ones I did in the hospital. Natural deliveries—whether in homes or hospitals—were involving me in a new way, and I was coming away from them considerably exhausted. It took me four years and almost two hundred natural deliveries before I could sit down for the labor and the delivery with the patient and her husband and come away from the whole thing without feeling emotionally drained. Slowly I discovered what I thought were the causes and the solution. I realized that some aspects of the delivery were for me and some for the patient. I had to work out which belonged to the patient and which belonged to me. Here is how it seemed to work.

Traditionally, we know that a patient forms an attachment to her obstetrician. From a purely logical point of view this should not be the case. A patient and her husband should hire an expert, and then use his services to help them do the things they cannot do themselves. That is because they do not know all the

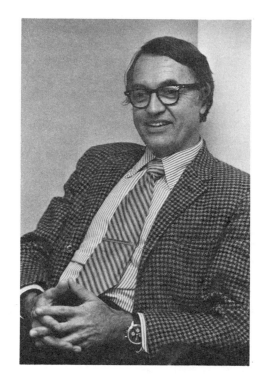

Dr. James Brew is engaged in private practice in obstetrics and gynecology with offices in Washington, D.C. and Bethesda, Maryland. He is a Clinical Associate Professor of Obstetrics and Gynecology at Georgetown University and on the attending staff at Georgetown University Hospital. He is also on the associate staff at Washington Hospital Center. Dr. Brew is a Fellow of the American College of Surgeons as well as a Fellow of the American College of Obstetrics and Gynecology.

After James Brew graduated from Cornell University Medical School in 1944, he completed his internship and one term of residency at New York Hospital followed by two years of residency in obstetrics and gynecology at Georgetown University Hospital. In 1952–53 he served as Chief of Obstetrics and Gynecology at District of Columbia General Hospital. The American Medical Association awarded Dr. Brew a citation for his gynecological surgery and obstetrical consulting in South Viet Nam with MEDICO in 1964.

intricacies of birth and need to have it made easier for them. When the birth is completed, the parents should then close the deal, pay off the expert, and send him on his way. Having evolved this approach, I decided the best way to proceed would be to teach the husband to coach the wife during labor, a task I had always performed before and which had involved me emotionally during my first natural deliveries. I realized that the husband could do it as well, feel involved, and that this allowed me the necessary emotional separation from the family process. I came to feel strongly that anything that would diminish the patient-physician attachment and encourage the couple cooperation would be a good thing. Since I could not find any literature on this attitude, I just had to work it out for myself and my patients.

From the beginning I thought that being present at a home would help create a more relaxed situation for everyone. I would be the expert ready to help when needed, but the location would be the domain of the patient, not that of the expert. In the hospital environment the doctor may feel at ease, but certainly the ordinary person finds it artificial and sterile. Hospitals just seem to be the wrong kind of atmosphere for what is essentially a healthy, normal, natural event. The home setting allows a husband and wife to remain the center of attention, thus reducing the isolation of the husband and the intrusion of the doctor.

My Philosophy

Let me explain a little about my philosophy of home deliveries. I view any project that a married couple enters into together as an adventure. I always viewed the classic obstetrician-patient relationship as one that separated husbands and wives. The doctor stepped between them. He would usually say, "Don't

worry about a thing. *I'll* take care of *you*, and *I'll* take care of your *baby*, and *I'll* take care of *things*." I wanted to stop that kind of thinking. The experience should belong to the husband, wife, and baby, and not to the physician.

There are milestones in every marriage. Meeting these milestones together builds a relationship. Deaths, sicknesses, and other crises are family affairs to be met and worked out together. Having a

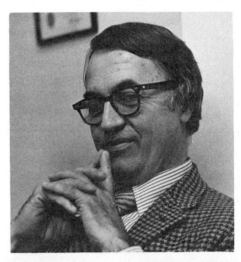

baby is the most important marriage adventure of all: it literally creates the family. Couples should meet and experience birth together and come away from it with the knowledge they've done it as a family. The obstetrician should help rather than hinder the process of making a couple into a family. And this, of course, is best done in an environment that fosters and aids this process, rather than in one that drives the couple apart. Natural childbirth at home brings the couple together in a close personal experience. What I have to offer that other doctors don't or won't offer is the setting—the couple's home. If all aspects of togetherness and natural delivery are there except for the home setting, then that's still better than the traditional

37

medicated hospital delivery. But the home is clearly the optimum setting.

To illustrate how strongly I feel about this approach, I have been involving the fathers of unmarried mothers in their deliveries. I've been asking the partners of unwed mothers to come in and take classes and be labor coaches and participate in deliveries. I'm not sure if this creates lasting values, but I sense that it's the best for all concerned for the time being.

One of the most difficult things to get across to young parents is that the trend toward hospital births is a new thing in the United States. In 1935, 35 percent of babies in this country were born in hospitals and the rest at home; by 1965 the figures were reversed, with 65 percent of babies being born in hospitals. In 1976 that number had apparently gone over 95 percent. There are still three large areas in the U.S. where births are largely handled by midwives in non-hospital settings. Kentucky is one, although I understand that the number of home births is declining. Another is in Arkansas and third is in the Indian territories of Arizona and New Mexico.

Overseas, the situation is entirely different. India and China, with most of the world's people, still have their births mainly done at home. In England, 35 percent of the current deliveries are done by midwives. In Norway and Holland the figures are well over 50 percent.

Is Home Birth Safe?

Without a doubt, the most frequently asked questions of me about home deliveries concern safety. I think I can put most of these anxieties to rest. In the first place, every woman who has a baby in the hospital has to travel to the hospital, whether she goes by previous plan or not. With few exceptions, almost all women who deliver in the hospital go

to the hospital during labor. Some go early, some go in the middle, and some, if questioned, would say, "I just barely got there!" Some women who plan to deliver in the hospital have their babies on the way—in the back seats of their cars. So, if anything did happen during labor at home that necessitated transfer to a hospital, the woman would be taking the same action as 95 percent of the other laboring women in this country.

Dangerous deliveries are almost all predictable. Neither I nor any other reasonable doctor would recommend a home delivery to a woman who was judged likely to have problems with her baby. About 8 percent of all births are considered abnormal or unusual and they are practically always known in advance. From the beginning, I only allowed my normal patients to deliver at home: that meant no breech births, no "bleeders," or the like. Over the years I accepted almost 600 women as satisfactory for home deliveries. Of these, about 560 actually delivered in their homes. The rest, about 8 percent, switched to hospitals for a variety of reasons. Most of these decisions to go to the hospital were made sometime during pregnancy; a few were made during labor; very, very few women had to go to the hospital as a last minute emergency. Of the home births, only one woman gave serious bleeding problems and had to be moved to a hospital at the last minute. There was one prolapsed cord, and the case came out well with a healthy baby.

Of all the patients I accepted for home delivery and delivered at home, I never lost a mother or a baby. This is in contrast to the average in the United States of about 1½ percent fetal loss and neonatal fatalities of twelve out of every one thousand births. Of course, the reason my figures were so good was that I accepted for home deliveries cases that I determined to be normal. Still, it is a safe experience.

One of the worries that women brought to me was a fear of infection during delivery. I guess this idea was either being read somewhere or passed down orally through the years. In this area, there is no question of the safer place for births. It is at home. Between 2 and 4 percent of the hospital deliveries result in infections. "Childbed fever" is indeed a deadly disease. The best way to get that at home is from either the doctor or nurse who comes to assist.

I suppose the other area of major concern is hemorrhaging. It is proper to question the statistics, but I believe they show there is no real need to worry. Usually, about 4 percent of the mothers in hospital deliveries do hemorrhage. That means they lose more than 600 cubic centimeters of blood. Because I selected only normal patients for home deliveries, I had only three cases of hemorrhaging.

All in all, I consider it safe to have your baby at home. Certainly my statistics bear this out. In certain ways such as infections, birth is safer at home. If you do have a bleeding problem, then it would be safer in a hospital, where there is blood available. But, as I have noted, the chances of this happening without warning are rare.

Practical Suggestions

Women often ask me about the difference in preparations for home births. Every hospital has a routine for deliveries. I have one for homes. At hospitals I usually order a partial prep for the mother. The prep—shaving the pubic area—is really a convenience for the doctor who thinks he may have to do a repair. It is just easier. In hospitals it is done by a nurse, and since it is in the hospital, it has to be done with a throw-a-way razor. Scissors cannot be used there because you would have to either throw them away or sterilize them after each use. They are too expensive to discard and sterilization spoils the edge, so the razor is the norm. Following birth, the prep results in women suffering discomfort, and it's all for the doctor's and the hospital's convenience. At home the prep is done by either the patient or the husband, so it can be done with scissors, thus causing less discomfort. I'm happy with that and the women certainly are. In both the home and the hospital, I ask the mother to take an enema.

Other things must be done to get ready. I give out a small list of things to have on hand. No emergency or unusual gear is required. I like to discuss the type of bed the patient has. A narrow, stiff bed is best. It is not easy to deliver a baby in a soft bed. We request a placenta-catching bowl and plastic bags for discarding. I also request a map so I know how to get there. Shoestrings—for use to tie the cord temporarily—are on the list in case the baby comes early. A plastic sheet for the bed is the only thing that costs any money, and that's only about $6. I also ask for a place for me to rest —while we are all waiting for the baby to decide to be born.

Medication

I get many questions on medication for births. Any drugs that the mother receives flow into the baby. Ideally, I guess the best possible thing would be for the baby to be unaffected while we give the mother what she thinks she needs. But that is impossible. Babies are affected by medication. I know from my experience in home births and hospital deliveries that I can recognize basic differences in medicated and unmedicated babies. The newly born unmedicated baby is alert, pink, and lively. Depending on the amount and type of medication, the baby from a medicated birth can be limp, blue, and very unresponsive. Medicated babies are not available for immediate positive imprinting from the mother, and this is an important problem.* When the baby emerges from one environment into an entirely new one, he encounters sights and sounds and people and a vast variety of experiences around him as he begins this life's experiences. But medicated babies miss what is one of the most important moments of their lives.

For years I delivered medicated babies in hospitals, as I was trained to do. Then, for twenty years, I delivered unmedicated babies at home. It was quite a different event: in the one you have drugged babies; in the other alert and sparkling new beings. Frankly, I do not know what the long-term effects are on each of these groups of children. Nevertheless, it's certainly reasonable to speculate that babies born without medication stand a better chance of continuing their lives as they began them, bright and fresh and alert and full of joy and excitement. But I know of no source giving any meaningful comparison of babies born of mothers with and without medication. The scientific studies are yet to be done.

The medication option is set by the hospitals. Every hospital is different and has its own customs and procedures. One hospital in Washington requires little medication for deliveries; another requires a great deal. The rest fall in between. When I have tried, in the past, to medicate lightly in the hospital that practices heavy medication, I have gotten considerable flack from the staff. Hospitals simply have to learn to be more flexible; alternatively, more families may choose to have their children at home and determine for themselves if they want medication. And light medication can be administered at home with no difficulty.

*See below, pp. 65-77 for discussion of imprinting.

When I do give medication, it is considerably less than I gave before. I try to point out the facts on medication even to women who ask for a lot.

Benefits for the Baby

To fully realize the significance of a home birth, I think it is necessary to look honestly at the tangible benefits to the new baby. There are many, and I believe that mothers should understand what they are when they are thinking about their new children. First, and most important, the new baby is kept in the family where it belongs, and is not torn away and separated. Hospitals, by their very nature, separate the father from the mother, and the new child from both. A hospital causes separation and imposes rules and restrictions that envelop the most natural act in the world with a stressful unnatural atmosphere. It turns something simple and direct into something artificial, stiff, formal, and generally unpleasant for the participants. No matter how enlightened the hospital, the new baby is taken away from its mother for part of the time. If you look around the world at other cultures and you look to mothers throughout the animal kingdom caring for their infants, it is not difficult to see the artificiality of the hospital condition.

Should Other Children be Present?

Two of my home deliveries were for the authors of this book. In both of those cases; their existing children were present for the new arrival. I have had children present for several other births. I believe that this is a family decision. If it works, then it is a fine thing. If it is forced by any member of the family, then it does not work. In those circumstances, instead of an educational or interesting experience, it would only be remembered unpleasantly. I always said to parents

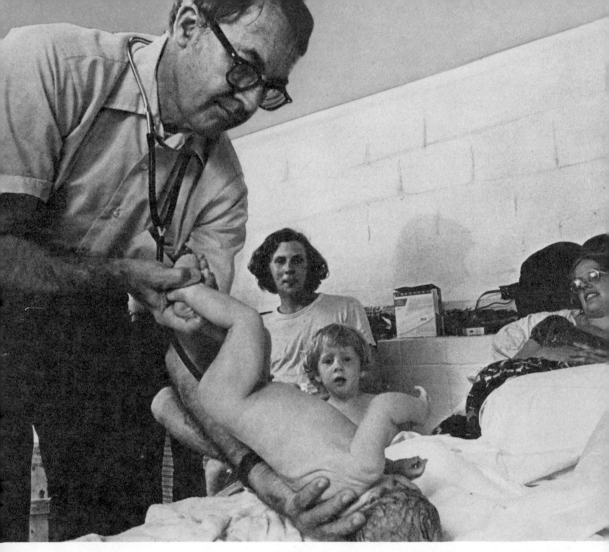

Dr. Brew examines the new Lamb baby girl as her brother, Jason, watches in wonderment. The proud parents, Jann and Mike Lamb, were still in the process of renovating their Rockville, Maryland, apartment when their second child was born.

that it was their decision. If one or more of their children wants to be there, then it is great. I have had no regrettable experiences. It is purely a very interesting episode in the lives of most of the children I have had around to watch their brothers and sisters being born.

Timing

I guess one of the most famous clichés in American life is the couple who call the doctor in the middle of the night, then race to a taxi or their car, dash toward the hospital, and have the baby before arriving. This kind of thing is completely unnecessary. Why shouldn't the couple stay quietly at home, with the expectant mother lying in her own bed, while the doctor drives to beat the baby's arrival? Naturally, delivering as many babies as I did, and not inducing labor so that the baby came on any schedule but its own, I had to have a system to get my own sleep and yet be present for the births. One of the first things I required of my patients was a map to their houses. That let me be ready. All my own equipment was also prepared in advance. I found that patients, particularly first time parents, were not especially good at predicting birth times. So the first thing I did was to send one of my nurses ahead. I then depended on the nurse to call me and tell me when to come.

Interestingly enough, I have kept figures over the years on some of my own arrival times at various homes. In a series of 55 deliveries, I was late for the birth 12 percent of the time, or 1 out of 8 deliveries. As it turns out, that is the same number of times that I and other doctors are late for hospital deliveries. That is because part of the time we get the call too late and part of the time we are just tied up on other cases and cannot get free to go then.

Outlook

At the present time, my home deliveries have been turned over to the care of nurse-midwives, who are certified and registered and who have had adequate training for the handling of normal obstetrics. These nurse-midwives are sufficiently well-trained to do prenatal examinations, including measurements, and postnatal physical examinations of both mother and baby. They are, in fact, *better* trained in obstetrics than the old general practitioners, some of whom still have privileges at the large area hospitals.

My present role has become one of backup to the nurse-midwife team. The relatively larger number of home deliveries being performed by them at this time is more easily handled in this way. My efforts as a specialist can be concentrated on the difficulties that sometimes occur in the management of pregnancies and childbirth. In the times when I was doing my own program, the number of home deliveries had to be rationed out, because I could only do a few. Now the nurse-midwives are able to do considerably more, about three times as many, or 15 a month. I am now actually supporting a larger number of home deliveries under the present arrangement than was ever possible before.

My wish for the near future is that there would be more midwives working. I believe that this increase would get the word out and circumvent the doctors who are unwilling to deliver at home and let more and more families have this experience. I guess what I really am hoping is that the market will create the suppliers. This is the classic free enterprise system and I see no reason why it should not work with baby deliveries as well as department store deliveries. If more families request or even demand home deliveries, then maybe we will have to have more doctors or midwives to provide the services. Natural childbirth is certainly an example of this. The market has created the supplier. Doctors generally will not discuss it but they were forced into cooperating with mothers demanding natural childbirth. When I started my practice in the 1950s no one did natural childbirth deliveries in the hospitals where I worked. Now, in those same hospitals, with husbands present, there are a large number of natural deliveries. I see this as encouraging. Something can be done and the place to start is to have a firm idea of what you want and stick with it. Shop around for a doctor with the type of reputation you want. Tell him what you are looking for in a birth experience and see it through. It is one of life's great moments and should be nothing less. I wish you good luck with all your children.

By Janet L. Epstein,
C.N.M., M.S.M. and
Marion McCartney, C.N.M., B.S.N.

In October, 1975, Maternity Center Associates, Ltd., became the nation's first incorporated nurse-midwifery service. Chartered under Maryland law, Maternity Center Associates, in Bethesda, is designed to provide primary health care to childbearing women, particularly to women who desire to give birth in their own homes. Janet and Marion, both certified nurse-midwives, practice under the general direction of two board-certified obstetricians, are partners in the corporation, and jointly administer the service. Our Advisory Committee is composed of an obstetrician, a pediatrician, a psychiatrist, and another certified nurse-midwife. This Committee meets regularly to provide general advice and to participate in quality assessment activities.

The Role of the Nurse-Midwife

We are registered nurses in the State of Maryland, and over the past several years we served as obstetrical nurses assisting two local obstetricians with home births. The day inevitably came when we "caught" a baby because the physician was unable to come to the home. It was an exhilarating experience for us. After a few such "catches," we decided to attend Georgetown University for the one-year midwifery course. Subsequently, we became certified by the American College of Nurse-Midwives.

The physicians with whom we worked agreed with us that the best way to satisfy the constantly increasing requests for home birth was for us to attend the home births as nurse-midwives. Nurse-midwives are generally concerned with "normal" women and in order to deliver at home, the mother-to-be has to be normal. This frees the doctors to practice their specialties, particularly with women who are high risks or who have complications of pregnancy. These physicians also act as consultants to our service in case we have problems we want to discuss. We have established a consultation clinic which is held several times a month. During this time, some of the supportive obstetricians in the community come to the office to consult with us on women who require special consideration. So far, our experience shows this approach to obstetrics is a practical and satisfying use of each professional's skills. Furthermore, it helps to fulfill a largely unmet need among expectant mothers. Since the medical profession has chosen to virtually ignore the public's desire for home births, we feel nurse-midwifery services can and should fill this void. Having our own organization affords us a sense of independence in caring for and assisting healthy women and their families. We feel that support and maintenance of optimum health is the unique function of nurses, and this is precisely our goal within the framework of our service.

We believe that childbirth should be a positive experience and that expectant parents are committed to doing what they think best for themselves and for their coming child. As professionals we adapt our assistance to what the parents want rather than attempt to convert them to prevailing medical philosophy. We believe that expectant parents have a right to give birth comfortably, capably and safely. Furthermore, we believe that a positive childbearing experience contributes to the development of a healthy family unit. Expectant parents have the

43

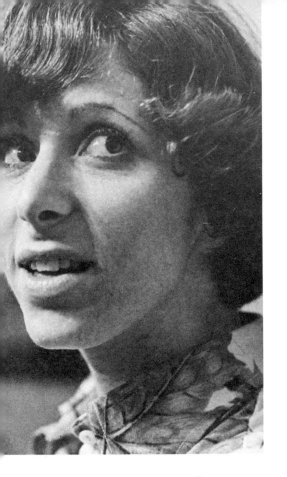

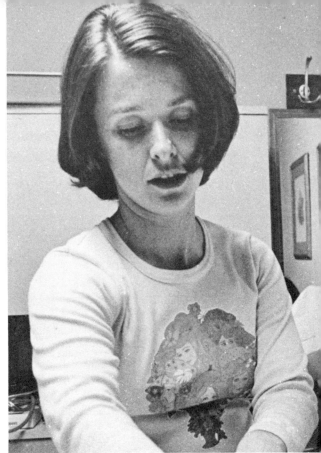

right and the responsibility to be involved in their own health care. Finally, we believe that cultural beliefs of the expectant parents should be recognized and respected. Occasionally this means that they question and sometimes refuse certain medical procedures.

In meeting the needs of those we serve, we provide comprehensive primary health care to childbearing women, including delivery at home for those who choose to do so and qualify as medically normal. We obtain consultations with and referral to physician-consultants or other medical specialists as required. Obstetrical clients are routinely seen in the office at a frequency of one visit a month up to 28 weeks' gestation, two visits a month up to 36 weeks', and then four visits a month up to term. Interpartum services are provided at home if the woman meets the selection standard, or in the hospital.

In the hospital, care is provided by the nurse-midwives and the physician working together, since none of the local hospitals allows nurse-midwives to conduct deliveries. As a part of obstetrical-gynecologic care, we utilize diagnostic services at two of the large area hospitals.

Teaching on an individual basis is an important part of our service. We give each woman specific instructions on how to prepare for her home birth, including emergency childbirth procedures. All obstetrical patients are encouraged to enroll in preparation for childbirth classes offered in the metropolitan area. We also invite the mothers and fathers of the newborns to attend a series of three group discussions centered on new family relationships in the early postpartum period. These groups are conducted by a psychiatric nurse practitioner who is employed by our service.

44

The history and laboratory results of each woman requesting home birth must be within normal limits. *Normal limits* is defined as no evidence of any of the following: hypertension, epilepsy, active syphilis, active anemia, diabetes, severe psychiatric disease, heart disease, multiple gestation such as twins, kidney disease, pre-eclampsia, abnormal vaginal bleeding, unusual or abnormal presentations or lie (breech), and previous C-section. Women accepted for home birth must appear emotionally mature and stable. Every woman is evaluated clinically (and by X-ray if indicated) to rule out cephalopelvic disproportion. Women accepted for home birth must have a completely normal, antepartum course. This means no evidence of the following: abnormal bleeding, pre-eclampsia, congenital abnormalities, inappropriate gestational size, multiple gestation, or unusual presentation or lie. Labor must begin within 24 hours of rupture of membranes. The fetus must be in a vertex position, and there must be no sign of infection. Any of the above abnormalities predisposes a hospital birth.

We try to arrange one visit to the home approximately two weeks before the delivery date. This gives the nurse-midwife the opportunity to become familiar with the facilities in the home and to discuss the birth arrangements in the surroundings where it will occur.

Upon learning that a client is in labor, the nurse-midwife notifies the obstetrician on call and proceeds to the home to attend the labor and delivery. After the baby is born, the nurse-midwife consults with the pediatrician chosen by the client.

During the labor, we encourage the client and her family to feel relaxed and in control. The woman eats or drinks as she desires. We see no need to restrict her diet unless she herself elects to do so. She is free to move about, use the bathroom frequently, and assume any position that is comfortable for her. The father of the baby, whenever possible, is the coach. He usually directs the rest of the family and is the major support to the mother. We do very little coaching, unless necessary, since the father and mother have been to preparation for childbirth classes and have hopefully worked out a system for themselves. If the father is not present, we ask the mother to choose a support person whom she cares for and who cares for her. As nurse-midwives, we feel our role is that of specialists hired to make sure all is well. We intervene only where appropriate.

No shaving of the perineal area is done. Rarely a small enema may be used if the mother requests it or if the lower bowel contains hard stool. We use no drugs of any sort during labor. If analgesia or labor stimulation is required, we feel this is best accomplished in the hospital. We do use pitocin, ergotrate and methergine, only if necessary after the baby and the placenta are delivered for control of bleeding. All procedures and medications used by the nurse-midwives have been approved by the consulting physicians.

The father of the baby is encouraged to assist us during the delivery. He can choose to be as involved as he feels comfortable. We have found that the overwhelming majority of fathers are eager to help deliver their babies and express pride in doing so. Family and friends usually surround the laboring couple and offer unique support. We encourage the couple to have whomever they desire to share this exceptional experience with them.

Episiotomies are done only if necessary, approximately 20 percent of the time. We repair them at home without difficulty. We do all we can to reduce the need for episiotomies, such as perineal massage and/or warm compresses as the mother desires.

Abnormal progress of labor can be treated with medical intervention and possible transfer to the hospital. The following situations require such action: elevated blood pressure, fetus in an abnormal position, meconium-stained amniotic fluid, fetal heart irregularities, prolonged labor using criteria established by Emmanuel Friedman, excessive bleeding, unengaged vertex in the primigravida with several hours of active labor, ruptured membranes over 24 hours, or, last but not least, the wishes of the woman.

The nurse-midwife stays with the mother and infant until vital signs are normal, the uterus is well contracted, and the baby is nursing well and shows no signs of distress. A minimum of one hour is always necessary. If any of the following should occur, medical consultation is required with possible transfer of the mother and/or the baby to the hospital: severe hemorrhage, retained placenta, lacerations beyond the second degree, or infant weight of less than 2500 grams (approximately 5.5 pounds), respiratory difficulties, cardiac irregularities, congenital abnormalities, Apgar score less than 7 at 5 minutes, prematurity, dysmaturity and postmaturity as determined by physical assessment. The pediatrician chosen by the parents is also available for consultation if a problem develops with the infant.

After successful delivery at home, the nurse-midwife completes and signs the birth certificate and gives postpartum instructions to the mother. Later, we make postpartum visits to the family to evaluate the condition of mother and baby. We see the mother at our office at two weeks and at six weeks postpartum. Family planning is usually discussed at this time.

There are a few lay midwives in our area who do home births. Occasionally they ask us to provide prenatal care for their clients, which we always do. Every so often during one of their deliveries, the client will have a tear. We assist the attending midwife with the repair. We are available to them for consultation at all times. We feel strongly that some medical expertise in these situations is better than none at all.

Our home birth service is very active now. Presently we do an average of 20 births per month. So far we are very happy with our results. Since the inception of the service a year ago, we have attended 180 families. Of these, we managed 143 home deliveries and 37 hospital deliveries (20 percent). Of the 37 hospital deliveries, 12 were Cesarean sections (6 percent), 4 were breech, 1 was a brow presentation, 7 had low forceps assisted deliveries, 11 had spontaneous deliveries, and 2 requested hospitalization for reasons other than medical. We have had one neonatal mortality and one mongoloid baby, who is alive and well at this time.

Positive feedback leads us to believe that our patients have been highly satisfied with the maternity center. We encourage these women to review their own charts and express their needs to us. This enables us to assist each woman in achieving the kind of birth experience she wants. We feel it is vital that clients be responsible for their own health care and contribute as much as they can to their own health maintenance. The service is proving to be a tremendous satisfaction and joy to us as nurse-midwives.

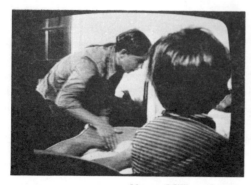
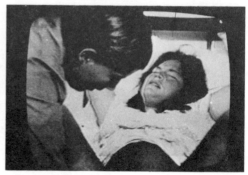

Nancy Mills assists in a televised home birth.

A Midwife's Story

Nancy lives with her husband and three children in a predominantly rural farming area in Northern California west of Santa Rosa. At the age of 28, Nancy has delivered approximately three hundred babies since she first became involved in midwifery five years ago. She works in a prenatal clinic called the Maternity Outreach Project.

BY NANCY MILLS

It was purely by chance that I delivered the first baby. I didn't even intend to be at my friend's home for the birth. I had just walked down the road and stopped to visit, and I found her in labor. She and her husband had planned to have the baby by themselves. I stuck around to help him deliver the baby. My experience with home births grew from there. Word got around that I had been very helpful, and in time another woman in the community said, "Since no one else here has seen a birth and you have, would you consider coming for mine?" So I went. At that point I didn't know if home birth was safe or not safe. I don't suppose I thought about it at all. I just went along to help out.

The third woman who asked me to help with her home birth actually had a lot more information than I did. She turned me on to some ideas and books. I helped her husband and her during their delivery, and it went on that way until I had probably done thirty or forty births. I began to study on my own—any book I could get—and with a group of midwives. With the help of a nurse from the University of California Hospital in San Francisco I located about ten other Northern California lay midwives and met once a month for an all-day study group. Doctors and nurses discussed pre-

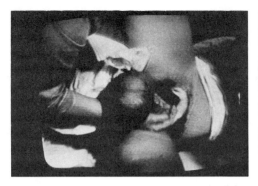 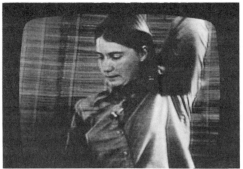

Courtesy of ABC News Reasoner Report.

natal and newborn examinations with us, and we shared experiences among ourselves and offered each other encouragement and support. The group worked together for about a year and a half.

At this time I met Dr. Michael Whitt in Point Reyes and his nurse, Helen Swallow, with whom I worked for a year. I usually went out first and checked on the mothers, tried to determine when the doctor should come, and called him. About 50 percent of the time he didn't make it until after the births, primarily because it was as much as a forty mile drive for him. I benefited from this experience, and he gave me the supplies I needed to have. After he went into partnership with another doctor and a nurse-midwife in Marin County, we stopped working together. They decided not to come to Sonoma County any more because of the long trip. After that, I was on my own for some time, but if I have a problem, I can still call Dr. Whitt.

My decision to devote much of life to helping other people with the birth of their children was influenced by my own birth experiences. I was only 16 when my first child, Tracey was born. Corey was born a year later. They were both born in the hospital with unprepared natural childbirth. I had an obstetrician who felt it was not a good idea to give me an anesthetic. He convinced me that childbirth was simple and that it would be easy for me since I was so young. And, in fact, it was. He was terrific. We had a big mirror; I experienced the whole birth by myself with no friends, no one holding my hand. I remember feeling very lonely. I had my second child the same way. Then my third child, Joshua, who's three, was born at home. My husband Barry delivered him. We did it ourselves with both my daughters present. The girls were seven and eight at the time. A friend who is a nurse was also there. It was really very nice.

In 1971 I began working with a nurse who had received a federal grant to study who was having home births and why. In our county, seventy-five miles north of San Francisco, there were many more home births occurring than in the city because many younger people had moved out into the country. The following year, 1972, we were funded again to establish a prenatal clinic, Maternity Outreach Project, which we are still operating. Since some people in our county live up to fifty miles from the nearest clinic or hospital, we meet a real need for them.

Maternity Outreach Project is a multi-purpose type clinic. We help with family planning, VD, well-baby check-ups, immunizations, and pregnancy testing

48

and counseling. If a woman comes into the clinic who wants to deliver at home, she is referred to a doctor who will support her. We discuss the risks of home birth with both her and her partner and warn them that there is always the chance that they might be on their own. Most families will not attempt a home birth without help, but some will, and I try to assist those families if I can. When I do attend a birth, I am not employed by the county or the clinic. I am acting on my own.

In the community there are five general practitioners who send patients to our clinic. We consult with the doctors, see their patients, and if we have a problem, they will back us up. None of these doctors will come to a home birth. There are no obstetricians who will even *see* a woman for prenatal care if she plans to have a home birth.

My original interest was in helping those people who planned home births on their own, but it grew to the point where I was supporting the community in home births and people were doing it because I was available. I have pulled back from doing ten or twelve a month to two or three a month. Today I just go out to those people who want to have home births regardless of whether I will go or not. Because I am working they understand that I may not be able to make it. On the one hand, I'm relieved because I feel those families having home births are making the decision on their own instead of my having that as my responsibility. I do feel strongly though that all people who want a home birth should have one—if they can get the help they need to do it safely. It's just overwhelming for me personally to try to give total help and support to so many; still, it's hard to turn anybody down. I hope the laws and attitudes will change.

Almost every woman I see has consulted a doctor. I also consult with him to see if he feels there's a problem with her having a home birth. I don't ever go against a doctor's advice. If he says, "I don't think she should have her baby at home," because of some specific medical reason, I say, "Fine." Then I try to encourage her to go to the hospital. On the other hand, if a person is seeing a doctor who I know is flatly against home births under any circumstances, then I usually recommend she change doctors. She deserves a doctor who will reasonably evaluate her situation.

If a woman is not coping well emotionally during labor, I just take her to the hospital. This has happened only twice, both times with women whose fathers are doctors. At home they were having prolonged labors, but as soon as they got into the hospital, they both had fine deliveries. I've always wondered if the reason was that they'd grown up with the orientation that the hospital is "the *safest* place."

I do not accept a breech presentation (feet-down) for home delivery, but I've ended up doing four at home. They can be complicated. One was a 7½ pound baby whose arms were extended over his head. It was difficult bringing one arm down and then the other. By that time, the cord had stopped pulsating. The baby came very slowly, so I resuscitated him and rushed him to the hospital. Everything was ok. He's three now and very healthy. Still, if the breech position is an established fact during prenatal visits or labor, I recommend that the woman go to the hospital. A woman who has had a Cesarean section or one known to be carrying twins is not a candidate for a home birth.

I am leery about accepting anyone for a home birth who is approaching her sixth pregancy. A lot depends on her past history. I did do a birth for a woman having her eleventh child. She was a Jehovah's Witness and refused to go to the hospital. She told me I could leave and she would still stay home and do it herself. If a woman is bound and determined to do it at home, as this one was, then I'm going to go to her no matter what her past history.

I do accept first-time pregnancies, including women with Rh-factor if it is their first pregnancy or later pregnancies if they have had Rhogam. I have been reassured by several doctors that usually there is time to get the baby safely to the hospital in case I end up with an unexpected Rh-problem.

If there seems to be a problem during labor we go to the hospital. I don't fool around with any signs of maternal or fetal distress; it's not worth jeopardizing anyone's life just to stay at home. Fortunately, out of 300 births, I've never had a mother or a baby die.

When a woman contacts me about having a home birth, I start by asking her to come to the clinic. We draw blood and send it to a lab for testing, take a history, and counsel on good nutrition and the benefits of prenatal care. Also, we encourage her and her husband to attend childbirth classes. Eighty to ninety percent do, especially if it's the first pregnancy. Childbirth Without Pain, a Lamaze class; Husband-Coached Childbirth, the Bradley class; and A.S.P.O. are all offered in this county. Before I had my son, I took two different classes so I am very familiar with the material in them. If a woman doesn't go, I try to give her the information myself and then I coach her through the birth.

Fifty percent of the women I see are on Medi-Cal, the state-supported welfare system. Forty-five percent are what I call "the working poor." There are a lot of gardeners and farmers in this group along with students and teachers affil-iated with the local colleges. I deliver babies for two or three wealthy women a year, about five percent.

I have attended some births in communes. At first I didn't know how I would feel going into them because of all the people present. The first experience was with twenty people. They were such a tight-knit group that they were in utter silence and awe over the birth. After the baby came out, I glanced about and noticed tears in almost everyone's eyes. Most of the home births seem to bring forth a great deal of love and affection.

Many families wanting home births are Jehovah's Witnesses, Christian Scientists, Seventh Day Adventists, and Buddhists. Perhaps as many as 60 percent of the families I see have very strong religious convictions. The atmosphere in their homes is usually very loving and, in many cases, they express their consciousness of God and His presence.

For the most part, families are well prepared when the time comes. Their homes are clean and they have bought the things on the list I gave them earlier. If I go into a really poor situation, I just do the best I can to talk to them about keeping themselves and the baby fairly clean. I do carry cotton and plastic underpads so that I have a clean surface under the mother. Also, I take along scissors, hemostats (clamps to prevent bleeding), a bulb syringe for suctioning the baby, shoe strings for tying the cord, a fetascope, a stethoscope, a blood pressure cup, a fish scale, silver nitrate for the baby's eyes and sterile water to wash them out with, Phisohex to wash my own hands and to wash the mother prior to delivery and afterward, and a stopwatch. I carry no pain killers of any kind, no muscle relaxants, no sedatives. I recommend that the woman not use aspirin, since it might increase the chance of hemorrhage; instead, I suggest she can

50

safely use Tylenol for afterbirth discomfort. I also carry instructions to give to her telling her what to do after the baby is born.

When the woman goes into labor, I go to her home. If it's far from my house, then I stay overnight with the family. I always try to be aware that the father should be the primary coach and the one having the closest relationship with his wife. I try to teach him to help his wife. If the couple needs some assistance, I massage or put pressure on the woman's back. I try to do all the little extra things that make her comfortable, like getting cold wash rags, ice, anything she needs.

I instruct a woman to deliver in the left lateral position. That way the woman's body is cupped around so she can watch as the baby emerges, and this position decreases the chances of tearing by putting the least strain on the perineum. Usually we put up a mirror. This is very helpful during the pushing stage. I encourage the father to help with the delivery, but if he doesn't want to, that's fine. Oftentimes, he delivers the baby. Then I lay it across the mother's leg while I suction it and dry it off. Then I wrap the baby in a blanket to keep it warm and hand it to its mother.

I've only done three episiotomies in the last three years. I only do one if it appears that there is no other way to deliver without a substantial tear. For the first two, a doctor friend came to do the suturing. For the third, he came and I did the suturing because he was teaching me. In the case of a very small first degree tear, I take care of it myself.

I do Apgar scores at one minute and at five minutes after birth. I've delivered two babies whom I rated 3 and 4. I've done a few that I've rated 6 or 7, but the vast majority are 8, 9, or 10. If I rate them a point or two down, it's because their reflexes aren't really good at one minute but are just fine at five, or because their color is a little bluish. Usually the babies have good respirations and heartbeats and color. If I hadn't had such consistently good results, I wouldn't still be involved in midwifery.

After the cord has stopped pulsating, usually within about two minutes, the father ties and cuts it. I explain the baby's interest in sucking and the benefits it brings to the mother. This stimulation contracts the uterus and slows down bleeding, so I encourage her to nurse right away. Then I wait for the placenta to be delivered.

In my experience, one hundred percent of the mothers breastfeed their babies! Many women are very much into natural foods here, and breast milk certainly fits into the whole scene. I'd say the shortest length of time a mother nurses her baby is nine months, and many go two years. One mother nursed her little girl three and a half years, only stopping then because she was pregnant again.

After the birth, when I'm satisfied that everybody's fine, I leave the room. This gives the family privacy to experience their joy together. I think the moments after birth are very important—a time to hug and kiss, to have a personal, quiet time. I know that this brings families very close together. Imprinting and bonding are experiences I have felt myself and have closely watched happen with families when the mother is holding the new baby. I've watched the father lean over and say something to the mother and the baby, and I've seen their eyes meet. I've watched the baby give a heavy look to the father and then back to the mother. This is an important moment and can substantially affect their future relationship.

I usually stay in the home for about two to three hours after the birth just to make sure that everything is ok. I return the following two days and one day during the second week, and I try to go back one day during the sixth week for a checkup. If the baby has a problem with jaundice, or the mother needs more help with breastfeeding I try to go more often.

If, during one of these postnatal home visits, I discover something serious, such as a baby's failing to thrive at one month, then I refer the family to the public health nurse or a pediatrician for an extensive follow-up. Sometimes I refer people to psychiatrists or child protective facilities, or whatever other resources I feel are appropriate.

I don't have a specific midwifery fee. Very often families ask me how much I charge. I usually say, "It's whatever you can afford." Often these families say, "Ok, fine," and they make the decision themselves. Sometimes I get paid; sometimes I get nothing. I try not to get hung up on money because my original motivation and my intentions were to help out—not to make money, I have a job working in the clinic, for which I get paid.

The personal rewards are what keep me going. I am very involved with the people I help. In contrast, I feel that the obstetricians I've dealt with in this county are on a money trip and have very little respect for women. Some of them refer to the women who go into their offices as the "mommies," which I resent. These men don't make home visits or even answer the phone in the middle of the night for a woman who is having a problem with a breast infection or with nursing her baby. As soon as the birth process is over, they seem to be very anxious to move away from further care of the infant. Their only thing is to handle the obstetrical care for the women, and the babies are expected to go to a pediatrician. I think serious obstetric problems should be referred to obstetricians. The family practice doctors, the general practitioners, seem to take a much greater interest in the family as a whole, because they are going to continue to be his patients.

A midwife can do a lot more for a woman and her family than most doctors. Midwives, being women for the most part and having experienced childbirth themselves, seem to be tuned in to all aspects of womanhood and its relationship with men. When it comes to revealing their sexual problems, their needs for birth control, and the way their children are relating to each other, women tend to be much more open with a midwife who has become their friend because she comes to visit. The women I help tell me our relationship has been supportive in many family-related areas. I know there are good, sensitive doctors, but my experience has taught me that midwifery fills a hollow space for a great many women.

By Russell J. Bunai, M.D.

A Pediatrician's Point of View

We all recognize the great joy which normally comes to a couple with the birth of their infant. That joy can only be complete, of course, if their infant is healthy. Good health ought to be the birthright of every infant, and healthy offspring ought to be the marital right of each couple. How wonderful it would be if these rights were realized at each birth and if each couple anticipating the birth of their child could be assured that their infant would be born healthy in every way. The health and safety of the mother and the infant is, therefore, central to any consideration of birth either at home or elsewhere. The question of prime importance is how can the health of the infant and the mother at each birth be most nearly assured.

Health at Birth

Preparation for health at birth should begin long before the time of delivery. The three stages of preparation are (1) preconception, (2) the prenatal period, and (3) labor and delivery. Preconceptional preparation includes protecting the genetic health of the population through public health and other protective measures.

Prenatal preparation involves supervising the health of the mother and safeguarding the infant from developmental anomalies due to maternal malnutrition, radiation, medications, or infections; it also includes the detection and care of any abnormalities of the pregnancy. The third stage of preparation for health at birth involves the skillful management of labor and delivery. This third stage, of course, is the one most immediately involved in the question of home birth.

Should All Babies Be Born in Hospitals?

In the interest of health and safety, should all infants be born in hospitals? At first glance, the answer might obviously be yes. Since the facilities necessary to treat the complications of labor and delivery are available in the hospital, the hospital might appear to be the safest place to have a baby. However, this is apparently not the case. In the United States over 95 percent of the infants are born in hospitals, yet the United States leads all other developed countries in the rate of infant deaths due to birth injuries and respiratory distress (neonatal asphyxia and other causes). According to the National Association for Retarded Children, there are about six million retarded individuals in the United States, and there is a predicted annual increase of over 100,000 per year. There also appears to be a progressive rise in the number of children with perceptional and behavioral disorders.

Since 1971 Dr. Russell Bunai has been engaged in private pediatric practice in Rockville, Maryland. From 1971 to 1975 he observed approximately 100 home birth babies in the course of his practice. His fifth child, Maria, was born at home in 1970.

Dr. Bunai graduated from the Tufts University School of Medicine in Boston in 1959. Following internship and service in the United States Navy as a medical officer, he completed three years of residency in internal medicine and pediatrics in Boston and Baltimore. As a medical missionary, Dr. Bunai worked for three years in Ghana, West Africa, in a general hospital that was the medical referral center for four maternity clinics serving a population of 10,000. His tour in Africa included wide experience in obstetrics.

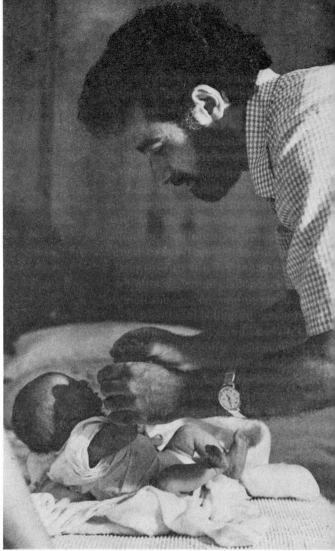

PHOTO BY CHARLOTTE WARD

Recent research makes it evident that obstetric medication, commonly part of the hospital delivery in the United States, plays an important role in this tragically high incidence of neurologic disability. Some 14 other countries have lower infant mortality and morbidity than the United States. Recent surveys have shown that Holland, where over 50 percent of the babies are born at home, has had the lowest infant mortality and morbidity.

Are these countries comparable, one might ask. Is the difference due to other factors that have a bearing on infant mortality, such as level of economic development, maternal diet, racial mixing of the population, etc.? Apparently not. In all of these factors, the United States and Holland are quite comparable.*

It is evident that the obstetric management of hospital deliveries we have come to expect as standard in our culture, often pathologically distorts an otherwise

*Many of these facts are outlined and referenced in an excellent report by Doris Haire, Co-president of International Childbirth Education Association; it is entitled The Cultural Warping of Childbirth, available through ICEA (See Part IV below for address.).

physiological event and increases the risks for mother and infant.

Should all infants be born in hospitals? It would appear that health in Holland would decline if there were a rise in hospital deliveries, and it would appear that health in the United States would improve if we achieved a greater percentage of home deliveries and a lower percentage of hospital deliveries. How could this be so?

Safety Factors in a Home Delivery

In order to better understand how home birth may be the safer birth, let us consider some basic facts. Health is a state of well being of body and mind. Health can be preserved or maintained with preventive medicine, but health cannot be created or dispensed by a physician or a hospital. Health is a state that can be recognized by the physician, but it cannot be improved by any remedy or treatment.

Illness is the loss of the state of well being through some physical, mental (or spiritual) malfunction. The primary function of the physician is the detection of any malfunction (diagnosis) and the taking of corrective measures (treatment). Disease, or malfunction, places the subject at risk. The correctly applied treatment corrects the malfunction and thereby removes or reduces that risk. However, all treatments themselves, especially if misapplied, carry with them a potential risk of side effects or untoward reactions. The use of treatments is justified only when correctly applied; in that case, the correct treatment eliminates the malfunction that has placed the subject at risk, and thereby, improves his state of health. Wrong treatment, however, increases the risk to the subject and is harmful.

Treatment of a healthy subject is wrong treatment and is usually harmful. In the case of a healthy pregnancy where the couple has been educated and prepared for a natural delivery, there is no treatment or procedure applied either at home or in the hospital that will improve the outcome of that pregnancy. On the contrary, the use of any treatment or procedure in the case of a healthy pregnancy constitutes obstetric interference and places the mother and infant at risk. Since obstetric medication, anesthesia, operative delivery, and hospitalization itself are treatment modes, these should be reserved only for those pregnancies where there are complications. The home environment usually insures freedom from obstetric interference in a normal labor. Furthermore, the home usually provides the optimal environment for childbirth. The importance of maintaining a comfortable and relaxed environment to the optimal progression of labor has been well established. Experiments have shown that when mice in labor are subjected to a disturbing, unfamiliar, or frightening environment, they have longer labors, more complications in labor, and fewer surviving offspring. Similarly, transportation of the mother to the hospital, labor in an unfamiliar environment, separation from loved ones, unfamiliar personnel and changes in personnel, attempts to accelerate or slow the progress of labor to accommodate personnel without obstetric indication all may have an adverse effect on the outcome of labor.

Labor is a biological phenomenon controlled by intrinsic factors but affected by extrinsic factors. With a home birth, conditions are usually best for a labor to progress undisturbed, on its own intrinsic schedule. In the early stages of labor there is no concern as to whether the woman is truly in labor; there is no concern about a premature or unnecessary trip to the hospital, or an unduly delayed trip to the hospital. In the early stages of labor, the mother may be up and about in her own home and may even eat and drink lightly.

Those familiar with home birth frequently observe that labors are shorter than average, more trouble free, and more joyful to the mother. The babies are typically alert and vigorous at birth with excellent Apgar scores of nine or ten. These results are due in part to the selection of only apparently healthy mothers with normal pregnancies for delivery at home. But this is not the only factor. When matched with comparable pregnancies ending in hospital deliveries, the home birth usually proceeds more rapidly, more easily, and more successfully for the mother and infant. When a pregnancy is normal and has been correctly diagnosed as such, and when the couple has been reassured of its normalcy and has been prepared for a natural childbirth and wants a home birth, the ideal and safest place for the couple to have its baby is at home.

Management of the Abnormal Pregnancy

It is axiomatic to the viewpoint presented here that the optimal management of a pregnancy that is not completely normal ordinarily requires delivery in a hospital. In the hospital facilities should be available to properly monitor and manage these problematic pregnancies with maximum safety for mother and infant.

Physical disorders complicate a relatively small percentage of pregnancies. However, a relatively common obstetric disorder in our culture is what might be called psychogenic dystocia. It has been well established that labor is a psychological event as well as a physical event. It is apparent that the difficulty a woman may have in tolerating the pain of labor is greatly increased by anxiety. This anxiety not only adds to the psychological burden but can significantly interfere with the normal progression of labor. Obstetricians like Grantly Dick-Read and Fernand Lamaze have clearly described this relationship and suggested useful techniques to allay maternal anxiety without the use of analgesics or anesthetics.

Since most couples are not prepared for natural childbirth, and since psychogenic dystocia is so common, lack of childbirth preparation itself ordinarily should be an indication for hospital delivery. Often in these cases, obstetric medication and operative delivery become necessary, adding to the risk of delivery, especially for the infant. The mother is usually unaware of this greater risk to the infant. In return for a few hours of comfort she may be risking a lifetime of heartache should her infant be seriously affected. Such a mother is somewhat like Esau of the Old Testament, who sold his birthright for a single meal.

Medical Personnel and the Role of the Pediatrician

The proper management of pregnancy ordinarily requires the services of an obstetrician, a midwife, and a pediatrician.

The entire pregnancy should be under the supervision of an obstetrician. However, normal deliveries are very well managed by properly trained midwives. Freed from the ritual of managing normal labors, the obstetrician would be free to concentrate his energy and skill on performing that service he alone is qualified to perform—the conduct of the abnormal labor.

The function of the midwife is to participate in providing prenatal care and to manage normal labor and delivery under the supervision of the obstetrician. Countries that surpass the U.S. in obstetric care utilize highly trained and skilled midwives in this way.

The pediatrician, ideally, should assume responsibility for the health of the newborn infant from conception. The midwife functions under his direction in the supervision of the newborn. Should the infant be perfectly normal, the pediatrician is not needed. In home births the pediatrician should be consulted prenatally regarding the safety of home birth. He should be immediately available for consultation during labor and for the management of the infant should that be necessary. In most instances a simple telephone call at the first convenient time by the midwife with a description of the delivery is all the postpartum consultation needed. Postpartum evaluation of the infant for the vigor of its suck, the sufficiency of lactation, and signs of jaundice should ordinarily be made by the midwife on postpartum visits during the early neonatal period. Any hint of difficulty calls for a consultation with the pediatrician. The pediatrician in some cases will be able to assess and manage the problem by phone; however, a home visit, early office visit, or hospitalization may be indicated.

Postpartum care of the infant could be simplified by expanding the prenatal care of the mother. For example, prenatal vaginal cultures for gonorrhea could make it unnecessary to use silver nitrate in the eyes of the newborn. Vitamin K given to the mother could obviate the need to give intramuscular Vitamin K to the full term newborn.

Preparation for Home Birth

Mismanaged or without adequate preparation, delivery at home can result in serious obstetric and pediatric problems. The properly managed home birth, however, is a significant advance beyond our present stage of obstetrics.

In order to be a true achievement and to enhance not only the joy but the safety

of delivery for both mother and infant, certain criteria for home birth must be met. In my opinion these criteria are as follows: (1) desire on the part of the couple to have a home birth and a desire to have the infant breastfed; (2) suitability of the home (The home should be clean, orderly, and hygienic.); (3) completion by the couple of an education course preparing them for natural childbirth; (4) obstetric care under the supervision of an obstetrician assisted by a well trained midwife throughout the pregnancy; (5) prenatal pediatric consultation and continuous postnatal pediatric supervision; (6) absence of any medical, obstetric, or pediatric contraindication to home delivery; (7) a trained midwife to be present throughout labor and delivery; (8) necessary equipment; (9) an accurate baby scale (provided by the parents); (10) a contingency plan in case the progress of labor is not satisfactory (This plan should provide for immediate obstetric or pediatric consultation, prepartum or postpartum hospitalization, and suitable transportation to a hospital.); (11) prenatal agreement by the obstetrician and the pediatrician that all criteria for a home birth have been met.*

Hospitalization After Initial
Home Management

Hospital admission either prepartum or postpartum should not be seen as a

*Some contraindications to home birth such as dystocia, placenta previa, or eclampsia are obvious. Others, such as mild elevation of blood pressure, which could predispose to abruptio placenta are more subtle. Other contraindications ordinarily include pregnancy in the early teens or in the older primipara, grand multiparity, onset of labor before 38 weeks or after 42 weeks of pregnancy, or a significant medical condition in the mother. A relative contraindication at any point in labor is failure of the head to be fully engaged; this might allow a prolapse of the cord to occur. Once the head of the fetus has normally engaged the pelvic inlet and the danger of cord prolapse is gone, this contraindication would then no longer exist.

failure of the home birth system. With optimal selection for home birth, such admissions are infrequent. There should be no hesitation, however, to abandon home birth and proceed with hospital delivery should any indication for hospital management arise. Postpartum hospitalization might also be elected. For example, should there be any respiratory difficulty or suspicion of infection in the newborn, hospitalization should be arranged promptly. In some instances, hospitalization for medical observation only is advisable.

Ideally, all hospitals would be organized and equipped for the admission of the mother and infant to the same room unless essential medical treatment makes that unfeasible.

Learning from Home Births to Improve Hospital Deliveries

In those instances where a hospital delivery is indicated, the total experience could be much safer, more comfortable, and more satisfying if certain physiological modifications were made in the hospital delivery along the lines of the home birth.

As with home births, couples should be educated and prepared for childbirth and lactation. The attitude of hospital personnel should reflect the fact that childbirth and lactation are essentially a normal process. The home birth experience bears out the fact that, when properly prepared and supported, the large majority of mothers can have perfectly normal deliveries and can nurse successfully.

Hospitals might consider introducing an "early labor lounge" where a woman in early labor can be ambulatory and chat with a family member if she desires. Home birth experience emphasizes the importance of a warm, relaxed atmosphere for the optimal progression of labor.

When labor has progressed to the point where confinement to bed is indicated, the mother should remain in the labor-delivery room on a labor-delivery bed designed for both labor and delivery. It is both disruptive and unnecessary to move an unmedicated mother having a normal delivery onto a delivery table or into a delivery room. As in the case of home birth, the woman giving birth in hospital should labor and deliver on the same bed in the same room.

A simple, firm bed meets all of the obstetric requirements for a normal home delivery. Similarly, the hospital labor-delivery bed should be designed for use with the mother in the semi-sitting position for delivery; it should have a foot-end extension to accommodate the new born infant. This bed, as with the usual bed at home, would have enough room so that the infant could remain attached to the placenta until the completion of the third stage of labor with the expulsion of the placenta.

Cord-clamping is unnecessary and hazardous.* Ideally the cord is not clamped at all. With delivery of the placenta the important physiological changes of this stage have occurred and

*Done promptly after the delivery of the baby, cord-clamping precipitates fetal-maternal transfusion which can sensitize the mother and place subsequent infants at risk. It delays separation of the placenta, and increases the risk of placental retention. Early cord-clamping deprives the newborn of placental oxygen which is especially hazardous in the asphyxiated newborn. With early clamping there is an increased risk of respiratory distress syndrome, especially in the premature infant; there is also deprivation of the physiological placental transfusion. This, in turn, predisposes to the risks of anemia and hypoalbuminemia which result. Proper management of the third stage of labor (from delivery of the baby to delivery of the placenta) eliminates these risks to mother and infant.

the labor has been completed. At that time the cord can be simply tied and cut.

Home birth affirms the togetherness of mother and infant. The mother and infant constitute a psychobiological unit. The early moments and the early days after delivery have far-reaching effects on lactation and subsequent behavior in both mother and infant. Of central importance to successful lactation is prolonged mother-infant contact and unrestricted nursing from birth. Failure to recognize this principle is a common cause of lactational failure.

Following a hospital delivery, the mother and infant should remain together in a "mother-infant recovery room," and rooming-in should begin promptly. Unless there is a clear medical reason for separating them, the mother and infant should remain together, as occurs naturally in the home birth.

Is the Modified Hospital Visit Preferable to Home Birth?

Many obstetrically well informed people are dissatisfied with the pathological distortions of childbirth that often characterize the typical American birth. However, they at the same time feel that home birth is an opposite extreme, and they would prefer an obstetric approach that avoids either extreme. If the hospital birth experience were modified and physiologically improved as described above, wouldn't we achieve the best of both worlds? Wouldn't we then have both the joys and physiological noninterference of family-centered home birth and the ready availability of medical resources to remedy possible complications of childbirth?

At first glance this might seem to be the best way of avoiding the two extremes. However, the fact remains that optimal management of normal pregnancies requires that no treatment be given,

while abnormal pregnancies often require hospitalization. Most pregnancies are normal, or with adequate preparation, could be normal. To require hospitalization of all mothers because of the much smaller number who require hospitalization is like putting all persons with simple "colds" on penicillin because a small number of them would benefit from penicillin. Optimal medical practice requires a precision of diagnosis which identifies those persons who have simple viral respiratory infections and should not have an antibiotic (Vitamin C in proper amount could be given) and those few who should have an antibiotic. So it is with obstetrics. For optimal obstetric management there must be a precision of diagnosis which identifies and separates those pregnancies which are normal from that smaller number which are abnormal and would require hospitalization.

When the diagnosis cannot be made with precision, the physiologically modified hospital birth is a suitable alternative to home birth. Such a delivery could be of the in-out variety where a mother and infant are discharged home shortly after birth if both are well.

The risk factor cannot be removed from life entirely. This applies to both hospital and home birth. Air flight does not come to a halt because of an occasional plane crash. The remedy for such accidents is not to abandon air travel but to work even harder to insure the safety of air travel.

The medical purist cannot escape the fact that in a properly prepared couple with a normal pregnancy no treatment is necessary or desirable and for such pregnancies the optimal environment for delivery is the home environment.

The Present Dilemma

In most places in the United States

today the medical community is not properly organized and prepared for home management of labor and delivery. Furthermore, in most hospitals in the United States today the medical community is not properly organized for the physiological management of labor and delivery. The couple anticipating the birth of its infant is therefore often faced with the dilemma of choosing between a pathological hospital birth experience or an improperly supervised home birth.

If obstetric care is to improve in our culture, we must make progress along the following lines: (1) recognize, respect, and preserve the essential normality of most pregnancies; (2) train and use properly trained midwives in the management of normal labors both at home and in the hospital, under the supervision of a qualified obstetrician and pediatrician; (3) refine the diagnostic selection process for delivery at home or in the hospital; (4) physiologically improve the hospital birth experience for those births not managed at home (Much is being done in this area in some hospitals.); (5) develop and perfect the medical system for the management of home births.

Hospital or Home Birth?

Until more progress is made in the development of the home birth system it is my opinion that all pregnancies should be delivered in the hospital except in cases where the essential criteria for home birth have been met. However, as progress is made in perfecting the home birth system, it would be preferable, I believe, if all pregnancies were managed at home except in those cases where hospital management is indicated. Progress in that direction would represent an obstetric and pediatric achievement of the highest order and would most nearly insure the health, safety, and joy of each mother and infant at birth.

In the last four years in private pediatric practice I have seen about one hundred infants born at home. In a few of these cases essentially all of the criteria for home birth were met. In most of these cases the most important of the criteria were met. In a few of the cases most of the criteria for home birth were not met. I was not consulted prenatally in the cases of this last group, and it was largely in this group that the small number of complications occurred.

While complete statistics have not been compiled, to the best of my knowledge and memory, the following is accurate:

(1) One mother was admitted to hospital prepartum because of unsatisfactory progress; she delivered uneventfully in hospital and she and her infant were discharged a few hours after birth.

(2) Seven infants were hospitalized in the early neonatal period; the indications for hospitalization were lethargy, poor suck, irregular or rapid respiration, jaundice, and possible or suspected neonatal sepsis (infection).

(a) Two of these infants were discharged after brief observation in hospital of less than one day.

(b) Five infants were treated for possible neonatal sepsis, but subsequent negative blood cultures cast doubt on the accuracy of the diagnosis of sepsis in all but one case.

All of the babies have done well and are in good health including the seven who were hospitalized. All of the mothers have done well and are also in good health.

So, home birth has worked out in practice and as a pediatrician I highly recommend it for the health and joy of the mother, the child, and the family.

By Miriam Friedman Kelty and
Edward J. Kelty

Miriam Friedman Kelty is Administrative Officer for Scientific Affairs at the American Psychological Association, Washington, D.C. After receiving her doctorate in psychology and psychobiology from Rutgers University, she did postdoctoral work at Clark University, Worcester State Hospital, and Harvard University School of Public Health. She has taught at The City College of New York, Clark University, and Boston College, and has consulted in the areas of psychology of women, ethics of research with humans, behavioral science and health behavior, and population psychology. Dr. Kelty is licensed to practice psychology in the District of Columbia and has published articles in numerous professional journals.

Edward J. Kelty, a clinical psychologist, currently holds an executive position at the National Institute of Mental Health that involves him in the relationships between mental health and other human service programs. Dr. Kelty graduated from McGill and Duke Universities, and is a Diplomate in Clinical Psychology of the American Board of Examiners in Professional Psychology. He taught for six years at the City College of New York and was a consultant in community medicine for New York Medical College, and has published numerous articles in professional journals. (The Kelty's own home birth story is told below, pp. 128-131.)

Psychological Advantages

The normal developmental stages of pregnancy, labor, and delivery have been defined by Erik Erikson as a "crisis" state, or turning point. Taken as a whole, these stages represent a transition for every member of the family. Either the crisis can be unresolved or poorly resolved and lead to psychological difficulties; or it can be well resolved and lead to healthy growth, development, and maturation. For some this change can lead to increased growth, inner unity, and the capacity to do well. Furthermore, the more nurturing and stable the environment, the better a new child can develop its own unique potential.

Home birth has been discussed from personal, historical, and medical points of view. Here, we are specifically concerned with the psychological implications. Since pregnancy is a psychobiological state, psychological factors heavily influence the outcome of pregnancy and delivery and affect attitudes towards and feelings about the birth experience and the newborn child. First we want to examine the stresses that may be imposed by hospitals in the United States today, then go on to explore data on the home birth situation itself.

Because hospital deliveries are now typical, many people are desensitized to

61

the erosion of human values that can occur with standardized care, particularly if the procedures are designed to accommodate sick people. The well-intentioned hospital routine often fails to meet the individualized human needs associated with childbirth.

Hospital procedures tend to counter the approaches taught in childbirth preparation texts and classes. This difference threatens the behavioral expectancies that prospective parents have learned and tried to use as their model for labor and delivery. Such institutional procedures may challenge the active participation in birth which couples now prepare for and anticipate with enthusiasm. The resulting conflict between what prepared couples want and what they get can prove a great disappointment, affecting how they view themselves, each other, their role as parents, and the infant itself.

Documented interviews and observations underscore the loneliness many women feel during labor as well as the lack of support and empathy from the hospital staff. Such experiences may result in depressive feelings and anxiety symptoms. One study of new mothers found that the majority had cried some time during the first ten postpartum days. Among the reasons they gave was the length of time they were left alone in the labor room. Another study found a positive correlation between the amount of touching women had received during labor and their capacity to mother their own newborns.

Of course, a hospital experience can be positive. It is important to recognize that an increasing number of progressive institutions are changing their obstetrical practices and policies to accommodate prepared-birth families and provide them with a more home-like atmosphere.

Frank Hatfield states the issue explicitly: "Should childbirth be regarded as a surgical operation, or as a great human event in which the whole family shares and which enriches and enlarges that family's experience?... All human achievement incurs risk, and in our efforts to reduce risk there comes a point at which the human value of the achievement itself can be destroyed."

The biographical sketches in this book attest to the fact that those couples who selected home birth after one or more hospital deliveries had experienced varied frustrations during hospitalization and relief and joy at home. They and many others like them have confirmed for themselves that birth is a time for the whole family. For an individual couple, home birth allows continued sharing of an experience that was initiated jointly and is apt to continue as a joint endeavor. Participating together in important events is a major factor in strengthening the relationship between spouses. Recent research substantiates what home birth families already know, that at home support can flow in all directions. During home birth, the entire array of family interactions is facilitated by the immediacy and closeness of sharing the event as it occurs. Greater privacy allows for freedom so that family members can express emotional support to each other in their own way whenever they feel the need.

For the youngest child, who is about to become the ex-baby, the birth of a sibling may be most critical. Fears of being supplanted by the newcomer make the event a potential crisis. At home, the parents and other family members have the option to keep all their children close-by, where the children can be held, and talked to and reassured. They can even be included in the birth scene itself to the extent the family feels is comfortable and acceptable for them. Maintaining this continuity of presence facilitates positive associations to the birth. Immediate familiarity with the newborn encourages more relaxed and spontaneous early contacts. Those children who either watch or are at least present in the home will think of birth as a natural process, rather than as an unknown, vaguely associated with hospitals and illness.

Only recently has the expectant father been shown to also experience a role change associated with pregnancy and birth. His participation and involvement help him to deal with changes he encounters. An empathetic and supportive male contributes to successful pregnancies and deliveries.

The familiar home environment serves to reduce tension and allow full concentration on the event itself without extraneous distractions. As the only one in labor, the woman feels secure in the care and attention she gets, and the new baby, when it arrives, receives similar special and loving consideration. In their own setting the couple is master. Others who may enter, such as doctor, nurse, midwife, have clear helping roles. Professionals interested in participating in home birth are sufficiently flexible that they do not require the authoritarian setting of a hospital for their own role support.

Home birth couples typically speak of their labor and birth experiences as relaxed and joyous. Research tends to show that home birth mothers have fewer illnesses or complications after delivery. This includes not only physical complications, such as tearing and hemorrhaging, but also postpartum psychological symptoms, such as depression and "nervous breakdowns," which appear to be virtually non-existent in home birth mothers. Most important, the home birth infant has been shown to be healthier up to a month after delivery.

Medications administered to the labor-ing woman have physical effects on her and the newborn and psychological ramifications on the whole family. A major advantage of home birth comes from the absence of medications customarily given during hospital labor and delivery. Until recently, it had not been scientifically established that these medications have behavioral effects on children. As a matter of fact, babies whose mothers were medicated during labor or delivery were found to feed for shorter lengths of time, ingest less food, sleep more, and be less responsive than those born to unmedicated mothers. An important new study found less rapid development of muscular strength and coordination, postural adjustment, visual following, and adaptation to sounds for as long as four weeks following delivery. The behavioral effects were proportional to the amount of medication given mothers during the birth process. Studies still in progress indicate that some of the effects persist during at least the first seven months of life.

What this means in terms of home birth is that the alert, awake baby is more responsive to and more rewarding for its parents. How different it is for new parents to hold a moving, wide awake visually active baby than a sluggish one who lies limply in their arms. How rewarding it is to have a newborn who immediately engages in vigorous nursing than one who needs coaxing or falls asleep instead. These very simple early behaviors are signs parents look for to indicate that their baby is healthy. The baby's responses stimulate a warm and exuberant relationship and lay the groundwork for positive interaction between parents and child.

Recent research indicates that newborns are capable of responding to considerably more stimulation than had been realized. They are sensitive to such maternal signals as eye contact and length of handling. They even make sounds in rhythm with parental speech. This mutual feedback between parents and infant is important in laying the basis for their interrelationship, which may otherwise be impeded by medications received through the placenta.

It has been documented that even within the first 24 hours, infants move their heads and smile in response to the human voice. Mothers consider it important that their infants look at them. Since both infant and parents influence each other, the home birth assures a positive climate where maximum learning can occur. It also provides the opportunity for significant people in the baby's life —mother, father, siblings, relatives, and friends—to share in developing these key relationships, as well as to deal with the life changes created by the event.

Three psychological variables appear basic to the decision to have a home birth. The first is the acceptance of childbirth as a normal biological process. This outlook is part of a positive life-long attitude toward the body and physiological processes. Those women who feel that bodily functions represent the "not-me" or "bad-me" are apt to worry about being sick during pregnancy, avoiding strain, and being generally incapacitated. There is a positive correlation between women who previously maintained physical activity and a lack of somatic complaints. They have less menstrual discomfort, backache, digestive disorders, fatigue, colds, and allergies. Women who are not physically fit are not as well prepared for the strenuous task of childbirth. The rapid physical and endocrine changes that occur during delivery will be less startling to those already comfortable with their bodies. The healthy acceptance of one's pregnancy and birth experiences is quite different from feeling helpless and approaching birth as an "operation."

The second variable is a life style that values sharing and joint participation. Couples who typically do things together will want to share the childbirth experience. Home birth requires a team effort. People used to being together so intimately are willing to tolerate each other's quirks. They are able to cooperate with each other in the intense situation of childbirth. Participating in the arrival of their infant becomes a shared peak family experience.

The third variable is the degree to which the couple takes responsibility for their own life experience. Even in a prepared, unmedicated delivery in a hospital setting, others are in charge and set the rules. In many ways, a hospital delivery is "programmed" so that someone else tells the couple what to do. For some, this is reassuring, and the hospital setting best suits their needs. For others, the choice of a home birth is still another facet of doing things for themselves. Home birth is a particularly satisfying experience for people who like to take charge of their own lives.

The psychological advantages of home birth include a heightened awareness of the experience through active participation, maximum opportunities for sharing, the familiarity and comfort of the home environment, and an optimal situation for initiating parent-child interactions. These are all logical extensions of the philosophy behind the prepared childbirth movement. Home birth provides the setting that most freely allows opportunities to practice the family-centered approach. The benefits of home birth and the growing demand call for additional well documented research. Establishment and circulation of such evidence will afford more families a clearer choice and a better chance of achieving it.

By Raven Lang

Raven Lang is the editor and co-author of the BIRTH BOOK *and one of the founders of the Birth Center, a group in Northern California devoted to home birth. She presently lives in British Columbia.*

On Imprinting

Recently there has been a great deal of biological research done on the effects of imprinting and motherly love among fishes, birds, and mammals. This essay is concerned with this type of research as it effects our own species, the human animal.

First let me describe what is meant by the word imprinting. It is a phenomenon which, because of an early experience, determines the social and psychological behavior of an animal. It is a word which Konrad Lorenz has popularized by doing much experimenting with animals of various sorts. To describe exactly what is meant by *imprinting,* let me use the following specific examples.

Example 1. Take a goose setting on eggs. When these eggs hatch, the goslings form an attachment to their mother and immediately follow and stay close to her. This process of imprinting takes place within a matter of minutes. Take another

batch of eggs and incubate them. When they hatch they will follow the first large moving object that they see. They begin to relate to this object as their mother. So complete is this process that if, after a few days, the goslings are given a choice between their real mother and the moving object to which they were imprinted, their choice is always the moving object.

Example 2. Take a turkey hen setting on eggs. When the eggs she has been sitting on hatch, the hen hears the chirping of her new chicks and is imprinted to this sound. The introduction of a stuffed raccoon (a natural enemy) to the vicinity of the nest will move the hen to fight it. However, if a tape of the chick sounds is hidden within the body of the fake raccoon, the hen will spread her wings and accept the raccoon as one of her own.

The first example of imprinting with goslings is one in which vision is the mechanism of imprinting, and it also shows how this process only affects the young. In the second example with the turkey hen, the mechanism is clearly one of sound and shows how it affects the mother.

With further exploration it was found that there is a critical period in which imprinting occurs, and with ducklings for instance, a rapid decline in the capacity to imprint occurs only 16 hours after hatching.

Miltown (meprobamate), a tranquilizer, was administered to mallards just after birth when they were normally most imprintable. The results indicated that with this drug the effectiveness of the imprinting experience was greatly reduced. It seems that some degree of anxiety is necessary for imprinting and with the interference of this drug, the normal amount of anxiety was reduced, thus affecting the mallards in their ability to imprint.

Much more research has been done in this area of imprinting, but I want to move on to interesting details directly related to the human animal.

R. Fantz did experiments with human infants. These infants were tested from birth to 14 days to determine what was most exciting to them visually. It was found that they preferred the human face more than any other pattern or shape and that patterns were of more interest than plain color. I feel the human face is preferred because it is part of the infant's survival, a recognition of one's own species: a social perception. Desmond Morris speaks of captive animals, which by mal-imprinting (being imprinted to a different species such as is done in zoos), have a susceptibility to becoming fixated on the wrong species leading to situations in which they find it impossible to adapt socially and sexually later in life.

My own pregnancy and birth experience and the experiences of women who

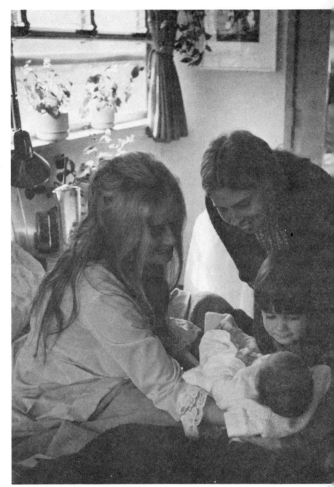

PHOTO BY JOHN BLAIR MITCHELL

Newborn children prefer the human face more than any other pattern or shape. Here, Stephanie Mitchell, just four hours after being born in the home of the John B. Mitchell family of Baltimore, discovers the loving faces of her mother, sister, and a family friend. "All my children are essentially happy," says Mrs. Mitchell who also has a son, Christopher, 5, "but Stephanie is by far the happiest. I cannot help but believe that her good-naturedness is the result of having never been separated from me at birth—having never to spend the first hours of life alone as most hospital-born babies do." Both Christopher and Jennifer were born in a hospital.

have delivered both at home and in hospitals are given here to demonstrate imprinting in terms of how it affects the mother.

In my own pregnancy, I remember reading that the process of involution in primates (the uterus contracting after birth thus causing its return to its original shape) began when the primate saw her young and heard their first cry. An example of vision and sound. I thought about this during my pregnancy. Imprinting causes involution. Far out. I wondered if that was why so many drugged women needed a shot of methergen or pitocin to contract their uteri.

Experience. Me. Stanford Hospital, 1968.

At the birth of my baby I was fully conscious. I remember a head rotating to my right leg and I saw a face in which I could recognize at least two generations of my past. A cry, forever imprinted in my mind, as clearly this minute as then. Heavy impressions. The baby was given to me for a minute and placed on my abdomen—then taken away to be wrapped and put in a plastic see-through box, far away and in back of me—so that I had to strain my neck to even see this little critter I had just parted from for the first time in his life. My perineum was stitched up and I was wheeled to maternity, my baby was sent to the nursery, my mate was sent home. I was to see my baby in several hours.

Each time the babies were brought to their mothers they would bring the babies first to the mothers who were at the far end of the maternity ward. I was in the room closest to the nursery, and so I received my baby last. Each time I saw him he was sleeping or quietly looking around. Later when the nursing shift changed, I heard the nursery door open and a crying baby being brought out to the mother. My uterus clamped down as it had when I heard my newborn's first cry. My breasts tingled and there was a definite gush of blood from my uterus which came from the contraction caused by the sound of the crying baby. When I realized that this was the first baby being brought out, I thought it must be a baby belonging to someone else and would be going down to the other end of the ward. But with another sound of that cry my uterus again clamped down and I felt complete bewilderment and a sense of demand for my baby. Within an instant he was being brought in to me by a different nurse. My body had known this child to be mine. My self was strongly reacting.

Had I been drugged and or unconscious, the information that I received at the time of birth would certainly not have registered as acutely or at all, and as a result I would have had less instinctual knowledge of my baby. I feel that when a woman first sees and hears her child at the moments of birth—which is another kind of consciousness—that she is bound to her baby already in a capacity beyond what I think we are willing to admit. I feel this is part of our survival.

Since that experience of my own involution, I have paid attention to the kinds of things women distinctly remember. Afterwards, most of them speak of that first impression as vividly as ever, and many are mentioned in the write ups presented in this book.

"The vision of that baby as seen through my legs will never leave me. Such profuse color, all purple and blue and red all at once, as she tensed expectantly in Pat's hands. John was about to introduce the syringe once more but in that second my baby burst forth in the lusty song of the newborn... I turned over and sat down. She was handed to me, cord still attached, covered with the yellow vernix, black hair matted in waves above her forehead. I noticed the molding of her head where she had presented and the swollen little flat features of her face. She flickered her eyes open and shut and proceeded to expel meconium all over my legs." Jodi

"It was an incredible experience to look between my legs, Kyle half out half in, first blue, then red and yelling, seems real hard to imagine anything more satisfying or beautiful." Doris

"That night I couldn't get to sleep at first. I kept looking at our baby—in fact that was my chief occupation for the next few days as well. She was just so new and perfect." Judy

There is one other aspect of the birth experience that I would like to mention, and that is the strange familiarity of birth. Birth is not totally an unknown or mysterious experience. A woman while giving birth has her own birth as a frame of reference, even though there is no conscious memory of it. The memory is communicated through the rhythm that the organism has already experienced, the same rhythm deeply rooted in the pre-consciousness of her own birth. I myself felt when actually in labor and delivery that I knew exactly the process, that I had always known it during my pregnancy and even before. Indeed, I knew so deeply the process of birth that when taken into delivery at Stanford and given a giant episiotomy which changed the time of my son's birth, that this was not the right time for him to be born. I remember saying to my mate, "This is not right, I am not ready yet." I remember attributing the memory of birth and the knowledge of it to the memory in my cells.

Stan Grof in his research with LSD frequently observed that female subjects reliving their own birth usually re-experienced on a more superficial level the delivering of their own children. He feels this deserves special attention.

"Both experiences were usually relived simultaneously, so that these women often could not say whether they were giving birth or were being reborn themselves. It seems that, during the delivery of her children, a female experiences an activation of her own birth memory and is able to discharge some of the tensions bound to it. This can be explained by the fact that both experiences have many similar elements and follow the same basic pattern." Stan Grof.

Now I would like to move to the birth experience for the baby.

We can assume that certain diet and behavior of the pregnant mother plays an important role in shaping the health and behavior of the growing fetus. And we can assume that the growing fetus does have an inter-uterine consciousness, the consciousness of its mother's heart beat, movement, rhythm, emotional experiences, sounds of the external world, and so on. The complexity of its mother's environment is its only reference point. This internal environment becomes one of ever increasing restriction during labor and with the child's birth this environment changes to one of limitless space. Otto Rank calls this the birth trauma. The infant at this time of birth is a complete sensor; using sight, sound, taste, touch, smell and rhythm. For the child, the time of birth is a period of great anxiety. Its world has just undergone some radical changes and the infant is feeling out for something familiar, something safe and gratifying. It seems reasonable that one of the best tools for reducing this state of anxiety is the presence of the mother. Here, with the very essence of this woman is the entire past of the child. Through the presence of the mother, the rhythms of that world and the security which those rhythms represent can be communicated. The infant should not be placed in a plastic hard edged box, isolated from the pattern of a human face, and denied the warmth and gratification that are her/his birthright.

68

In birds we have already considered that a sense of anxiety is necessary for imprintibility. This anxiety in humans may be related to the anxiety of being left alone. And anxiety is the mechanism which needs to be well functioning in order for complete imprintability. However, if the anxiety is kept going too long, it becomes more of a trauma than would be natural, and too traumatic an experience may no longer be valuable, but may even prove to be harmful. If we paid attention to the instinct of undrugged mothers we would give them their babies, which they so commonly demand.

And so, if this anxiety has a function, then the moments and hours after birth should not be condusive to increasing this anxiety, but toward reducing it through gratification. Adult behavior that is often anxiety ridden may in fact be directly related to a specific separation of mother and child at birth.

Effects of maternal separation and deprivation in the human have scarcely been investigated. We say we do not scientifically *know* the importance of these first few hours and days after birth for both the mother and child. (With time and research, the consideration must also include the father and the possibility of family and friends). We say we do not scientifically *know* to what extent we are interfering with natural functions when we separate the mother and baby.

Experiments at the University of Cornell engaged in a program of research for the prevention of mental illness using sheep and goats. They demonstrated the ability of a mother to protect her offspring from environmental stress by placing twin kids in identical rooms, the only difference being that one kid was in the presence of its mother and the other kid was left alone. An artificial stress environment was created by turning off the lights every two minutes and applying a brief shock to each goat's foreleg. After the goats had been conditioned in this manner they were tested two years later by exposing them to the same environment for twenty days. The goats who had had their mothers with them during their early experience showed no evidence of abnormal behavior in response to the severe stress of this environment. The others exhibited definite neurotic behavior. Somehow the mother's presence alone protects the baby goat from the traumatic influences of the rigid pattern of tensions to which the twin in the adjoining room succumbs.

If birth is to be regarded as a trauma in which stress is either created by the compression of birth itself, or the anxiety of the organism being thrust into a completely unfamiliar environment, then the importance of the continuous presence of the mother as a means of negating the effects of this stress must not be overlooked. It is interesting to note that as a part of related experiments, conditioned neurotic sheep or goats were found incapable of dealing with the situation of actual danger in realistic fashion, making their survival rate significantly less. This is because the animal's gregariousness is damaged and while other members of the herd escape together, the neurotic animal flees in panic by itself.

In light of the implications of these experiments with animals, the concept of natural home birth having importance to research in the preventive mental health field should be examined. The possibility that our hospitals through a gross oversight (as was once done with puerperal fever) may be contributing to adult neuroses through our present day rituals of birth should be looked at with much more emphasis than is done at this time. Could the separation of the baby from its mother be related to a sense of non-acceptance later in life?

The data on material like this in terms of humans is lacking, but it is coming fast. Scientists and psychologists alike feel that the infant's love for its mother is learned through association with the mother's face, smell, sound, etc., as well as her gratification of such needs as hunger and discomfort. Nursing, contact, and even hearing and seeing are also considered important in the development of the infant's love for its mother. All of these contribute to the development of the intense, loving, and profound relationship possible between the mother and child.

"The first love of the human infant is for his mother. The tender intimacy of this attachment is such that it is sometimes regarded as a sacred or mystical force, an instinct incapable of analysis. No doubt such compunctions, along with the obvious obstacles in the way of objective study, have hampered experimental observation of the bonds between child and mother." Harlow.

Other experiences demonstrate the importance of maternal contact at early ages in developing a pattern of affection in the child's social behavior, as opposed to maternal deprivation leaving it less able to form lasting ties. We know also that a child having physical contact has a greater capacity for handling stress than one who hasn't been touched, and that the ability to handle stress is directly related to shaping the personality of the adult.

"Investigations concerned with maternal deprivation report that children raised in foundling homes develop at a retarded rate and are more susceptible to disease." Levine.

This last section of the paper is primarily made up of comments from mothers about the experience of birth, and my own observations and thoughts on the subject.

Joan is a 19 year old woman whom I met in her seventh month of pregnancy. She had been married but was no longer living with her husband.

One day I heard a friend ask Joan what sex she felt her baby would be. Joan said it had better be a girl, and if it wasn't she would flush him down the toilet. On another occasion she said she very much wanted a girl. Some days later in conversation Joan told me that her husband wanted the baby if it was a boy but didn't care to have it if it was a girl.

At her birth which was two weeks after her statement of female preference, she gave birth to a baby boy. When she first turned around to get him, and had the sound of someone's voice ring in her ear, "It's a boy," I felt she was suffering from a disappointment that was real. At any rate, Joan proceeded to hold, examine, touch, talk to, nurse, and respond to her baby. It was the getting-to-know-you baby time and all the gestures that go along with it. Within one half hour Joan said, "You know, it doesn't really make any difference if it's a boy or a girl." And even later she said something to the effect, "It's not really in-born, this boy/girl stuff. Babies are really all the same and it's only society that makes such changes and puts such things on the sexes." And later yet, "I will not be sexist to my son."

The next day someone came by after just having visited Joan and said she was looking beautiful, and was a beautiful mother, full of pride and love for her baby.

Now my reason for mentioning all this is to examine what might have been Joan's feeling if she had been drugged and/or separated from her baby. Would her acceptance and insights and love have been the same? And would her son's separation have increased his anxiety level? And then after returning to his

70

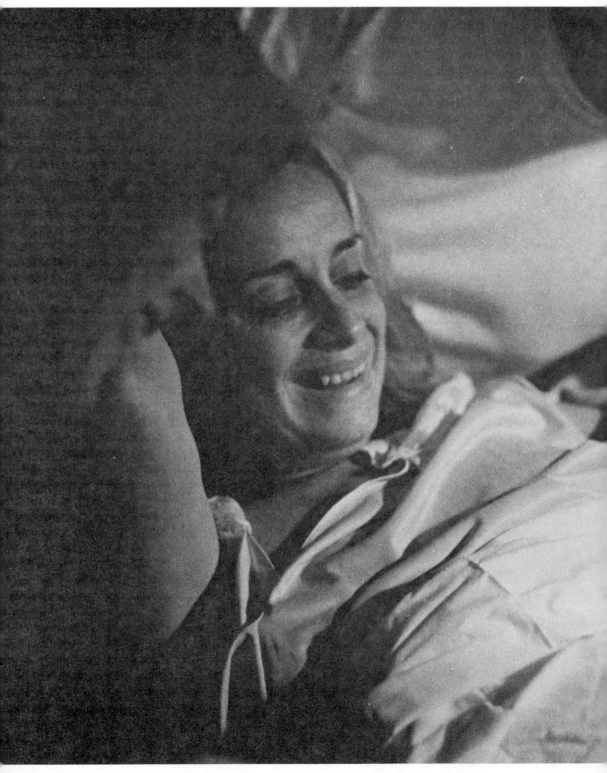

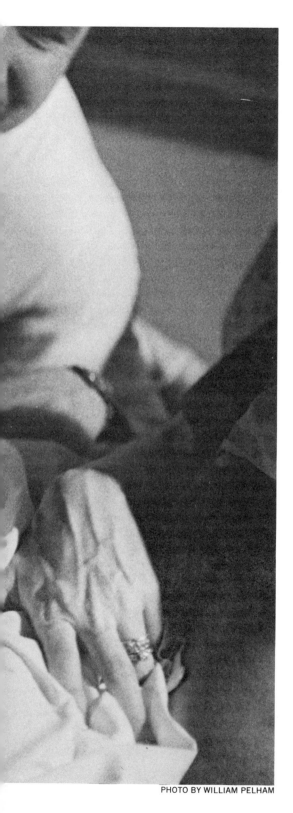

PHOTO BY WILLIAM PELHAM

The inter-uterine environment just prior
to birth is extremely
important for the child's future
psychological well-being. "It was
so nice to spend this labor lying quietly,
chatting on our own bed,
says Mrs. Mitchell. "I am sure it made
it an easier labor on the
baby, and it certainly was more fun for
me to stay home."

At the moment of birth, the newborn
infant is a complete sensor,
using sight, sound, touch, and smell
to seek out something familiar,
safe and gratifying in the new
environment. "What a mind blowing
sight it was," continues Mrs. Mitchell.
"I was delighted to feel
her tiny hand reaching up on my leg when
she was only seconds old.
We shouted in surprise, for the
predictions were for a boy. I was
able to see everything perfectly in the
soft light, unencumbered by
the pounds of sterile hospital sheets.
This definitely was the way
to have a child!"

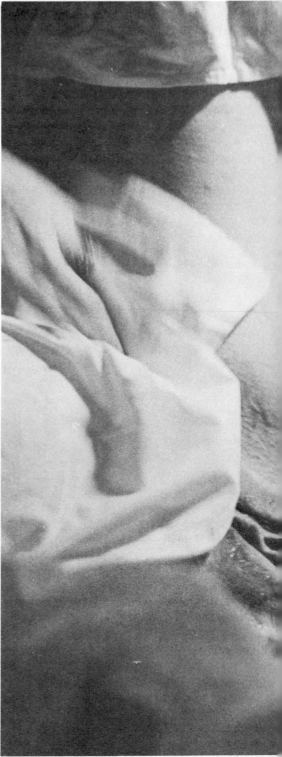

PHOTO BY WILLIAM PELHAM

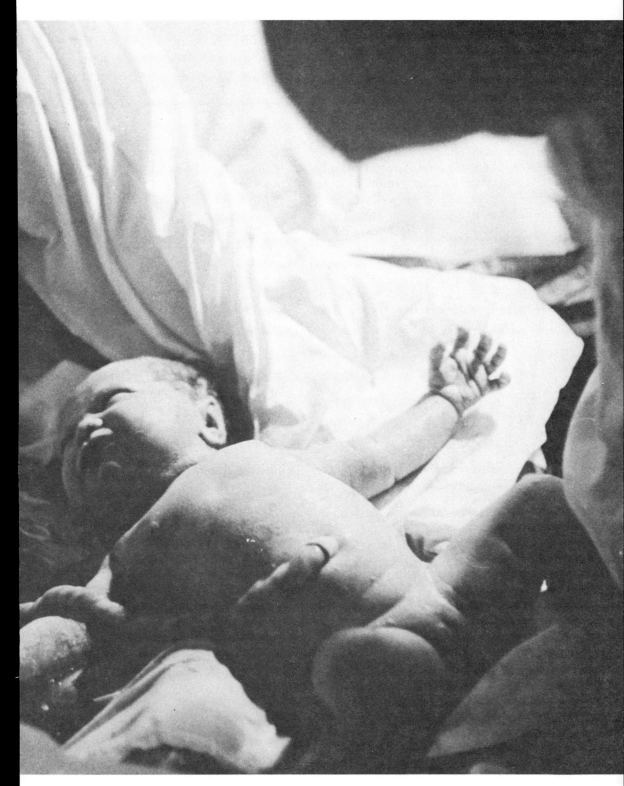

mother five to 12 hours later, would he have felt the beginnings of non-acceptance and rejection, which may by routine separation be increased? We do know that when a goat kid or calf is removed from its mother at birth, and returned some hours later, there may be maternal rejection, even to the point of death for the young.

Another example: Approximately three years ago a friend of mine became pregnant. She tried to find a doctor from Santa Cruz to Berkeley who would help her have her baby at home, but she could get no one to help her. The most agreeable thing to her was to go to San Francisco's French Hospital, where the LaMaze method of birth was in common practice. Her labor was fairly fast and easy. Her husband was allowed to witness the birth, and all in all she had a very positive hospital birth. However, minutes after her baby was born he was wisked out of the room and sent to the nursery for six hours. The nursing routine was to bring the babies to the mother every four hours for fifteen to twenty minutes.

Just a month ago, this woman came to our home birth seminar and told the attending group the story of her birth. She described the post-birth experience at the hospital as the most painful thing she has experienced in her life. She told us of the four-hour periods when her son would be in the nursery, crying and crying, and how she stood on the other side of the window and also cried and cried. But her baby remained in the nursery and she on the other side of the glass. She also mentioned her sorrow that at this time she didn't simply demand her baby or physically get him and go home. But because of the vulnerability of her birth state, and her ignorance of the laws governing her, this did not happen. This incidence turned what should have been

one of the highest experiences of her life into the most painful, and I question the results of that kind of interference. This is not to say that all women and/or babies are as hurt by this event, but we should not assume all women and/or babies to be unaffected.

A unique experience of imprinting beyond the mother and child occurred at the birth of Trava. There was a group of eleven people at this birth. In the first two hours of Trava's extra-uterine life, he was passed around from member to member of his family, all of whom were deeply moved. It was an extremely high intensity vibration birth. I, myself, felt part of this family, a kind of we-have-known-each-other-for-a-long-time-already feeling.

One day, only weeks after Trava's birth, his parents and family were all in one room quietly sitting when he rolled off the chair and onto the floor. Emily, his mother, in recounting this story told me that Gary, a member of the family and present for the birth, reacted and looked exactly as she herself felt and acted, and he looked and responded in the same manner and intensity and speed as Harry had done. (Harry being the natural father). When telling me this story Emily expressed a feeling and statement and this is a quote, "As Harry is Trava's father, and I his mother, also Gary is his father." Emily, Harry, and Gary did not fully understand this link, or how it came to be.

This kind of experience happens to varying degrees all the time at home birth. Bertrand Russell speaks of this multiple parent phenomenon amongst Trobriand Islanders who give birth in tribal situations. The most recent experience I had involving this issue happened two weeks ago at the Birth Center. There were two newborns present on this day. One of the newborn's births I had attended, and the other I had not. Both of the babies were put side by side and we were looking at them together. The experience of my observation of the baby whose birth I had not attended was beautiful, healthy, full term looking baby, while the feeling I had for the other baby was of tremendous closeness to him. I felt a bond with him. This is the bond of birth which I am talking about, the same bond that affected Gary so strongly.

I would like to conclude with a few observations concerning the home birth ceremony that I have witnessed time and again at the deliveries I have attended.

The child usually quiets down when given to the mother. She/he seems to be sensing the lights of this world, its sounds, smells, air, a new sense of freedom of movement, and so on. Almost always, the baby looks good and hard at the mother, and the mother is usually glued to the splendor of her baby. Usually the mother rubs the baby's skin, starting with the face. The rubbing is done with the mother's fingertips and is always a very gentle stroking motion. I believe this is the first natural gesture made by the mother, and not necessarily the beautiful act of nursing. The baby is usually offered a nipple, but often doesn't suck right away. The most common action for the baby when given a nipple is to lick the mother's nipple over and over. I believe the infant is also smelling the mother. The infant has no trouble knowing the breast, and that it is a source of food. The baby's instinct is always to turn her or his head in the direction of the offered nipple. I feel what the mother is saying to her baby is also being recorded. If the baby is with the mother for some time after birth, and then passed to someone else, the behavior of the child will be to cry and fuss in the arms of another. When the infant is returned to the mother, she or he will almost always quiet down and begin to like her nipple if it is near and available. It looks to me that the infant already knows its mother and is bound to her deeply.

If there is anything valid in home birth beyond a couple's right to be free to choose the manner in which their child shall be born, it is in the areas of imprinting, where the mother's love as well as the love of all present, are important in the developing relationship between the child and these people, as well as the child's own sense of self-love.

These are some of my arguments for home birth. A midwife would most likely be more sensitive to the woman's emotional and physical state, and for this reason she would be better suited to work with the woman if she were well trained. She would be able to stay with both the mother and child for several hours after birth unlike the professional is willing to do. Mother would do more following of her own instincts as would baby. Midwives can be trained to make and record observations concerning the birth. Records can be kept during pre- and post natal care of diet, emotional state, and the life style and environment in which the mother and fetus live. All of this information could be used in studying the relationship between birth and neurosis.

And so we question. We ask ourselves about ourselves in order to understand ourselves better and to correct the sometimes brutal yet seemingly innocent things that have been done to us, in order for us not to do them to our own children. A simple quest for bettering the future.

By Patricia Nicholas

The Lasting Impact

We are all born needing. Our basic needs are not excessive. They are the central reality of the infant. These needs are: to be fed, to be kept warm and dry, to grow and develop at our own pace, to be held and caressed, to be stimulated, and to be allowed to express ourselves. To an infant this means he is loved. The only way to guide a baby toward mental health, the only way to nurture a feeling child, is that which derives from the knowledge of the baby's own biological and psychological realities.

The topic of home birth usually brings the question, "But is it safe?" Obviously the reference is to the infant's physical health, but his psychological health is just as important. In my work, I deal with neurotic adults whose neuroses are sometimes brought on by their own bad birth experiences. To avoid these problems in today's infants, I am recommending calm, drug-free, natural births in a relaxed atmosphere. Such deliveries are most likely to occur in the familiar and supportive environment of the home.

Many people who study births have noticed that there are differences between babies right from delivery. I often follow the progress of babies, and I see that the basic personality traits that derive from the nature of their birth do not drastically change later on. A. S.

Neill, the famous educator, wondered in his book *Summerhill* why one baby is born with a shrinking soul and another with courage; Neill concluded that this was probably due to prenatal conditions and a mother's transference of anxiety or gladness.

By using a clapper and a vibrator, Dr. D. K. Spelt illustrated in 1948 that fetuses *in utero* would react with great activity when a programmed series of noises and vibrations were executed. In this classic example of conditioned response, it was demonstrated that fetuses actually learned in the womb. If a baby can learn in the womb, I believe that a baby can also *feel* in the womb, by which I mean he can experience and know the sensations of fear, alarm, frustration, etc.

All neurotic people are fraught with a common characteristic—that of tension. Neurotic tension is the by-product of either physical or psychological pain. A person's history of pain builds until it reaches a point when that person builds a set of defenses that obscures reality. Primal Therapy, the field in which I work, systematically dismantles these defenses and thereby enables the person to relive his original early hurts. After the reliving (called a Primal) a person can connect the old feeling that he experienced to his present life and interpret its meaning to him, giving him new and lasting insight. It is this process which throws over the person's repression and neurotic symptoms and helps him to find his real self, his natural impulses and feelings.

Many of the Primals that people experience in therapy are the reliving of the conditions of their pregnancies, births, and early hours afterwards. My work with adults reliving their birth experiences indicates that unfortunate occurances and medical interference caused pains and traumas that have accompanied these people throughout their lives.

While many seem to consider a baby "undeveloped to the point of being unconscious," I recognize a baby as an acutely conscious and vulnerable human being who is totally capable of experiencing any pain, hardship, deprivation, or insult to his person, to such a degree, in fact, that early trauma can be responsible for prototypic behavior that will characterize the person for a lifetime. If the pain is great enough, the baby may have to split off from it and thus from himself. If not, it can be the beginning of a series of pains that, when accumulated, will have to be repressed for a lifetime or reexperienced in therapy.

When does a baby begin to feel? The baby is originally nurtured in a womb where he can hear the warm gurglings and the familiar heartbeat of his mother. As early as five months after conception the baby develops a consciousness, an awareness, if you want to call it that. How do we know? Because he can begin to respond to touch and sound. It is my belief that faulty mother-child relationships—and so neurosis—can have prenatal origins. Babies may even sense whether they are wanted or not.

With the understanding that fetuses and newborns are aware, the importance of a good birth experience becomes evident. An infant is so fragile, so unprotected, so helpless, and so totally at the mercy of his environment that for him to undergo abnormal birth conditions can cause or contribute to neuroses that will last throughout his adult life. It is my conviction that human anxiety and unhappiness can be lessened by recognizing and meeting the emotional needs of the infant from the beginning. This is precisely the reason I support home births and have also designed and instructed a Childbirth Education Association class especially for home birth couples.

The home automatically provides the

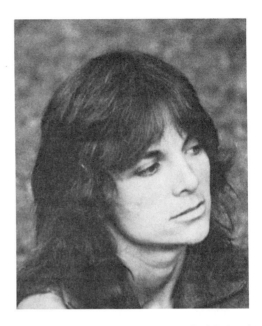

Patricia Nicholas is a certified Primal Therapist and an executive board member at the Primal Institute. She works in an Antioch College graduate studies program in Clinical Psychology in conjunction with the Primal Foundation for Research and Education.

Her textbook, Labor of Love, *is widely used by childbirth educators. She addressed the Childbirth Education Association of Los Angeles on "Humanistic Childbirth To Make Whole Persons." Her paper, "Childbirth—Does It Have To Be Painful?", appears in Dr. Arthur Janov's book,* The Anatomy of Mental Illness. *Another paper, "From Womb to World," was published in* The Journal of Primal Therapy.

Ms. Nicholas not only writes about humanistic childbirth; she works to further the practice. She was certified as a Childbirth Educator by The American Institute for Family Relations in Los Angeles, and has taught special classes for home births. Ms. Nicholas lives with her husband and two children in Sherman Oaks, California.

best opportunity for a relaxed birth without the tenison and interference often accompanying hospital deliveries. However, today's obstetric skills and knowledge are too precious to forego. I do not endorse professionally unattended births. The shortage of available and interested doctors who will deliver at home is a great problem in some areas of the country. With the development of a proper system of trained midwives and emergency mobile birth units, many normal women who have received adequate prenatal care and desire to give birth at home can safely do so.

Virtually all medications interfere with a baby's chances for a healthy survival. Besides the physical handicaps with which the baby has to contend, he may further act out his birth Primal for the rest of his life. One Primal patient connected his "deadness," his inability to respond spontaneously, to being numbed from birth by the use of drugs.

In a home delivery the mother gets a good deal of psychological and emotional support, the ingredients that Dr. Donald M. Sherline, a practicing obstetrician in Jackson, Mississippi, feels are necessary to avoid the use of routine anesthesia. Speaking at a meeting of The American College of Obstetricians and Gynecologists, he argued that the demand for anesthesia was largely cultural and that if women were informed accurately as to the consequences of the anesthesia offered, they would use psychoprophylaxis techniques and opt for an unmedicated birth.

At the same meeting Dr. Abner Levkoff of the Medical University of South Carolina said that if anesthesia were reduced in this country, the problem of newborn infant resuscitation would be less acute. He stated that about 5 percent of term babies delivered vaginally with no serious disease are born limp or with-

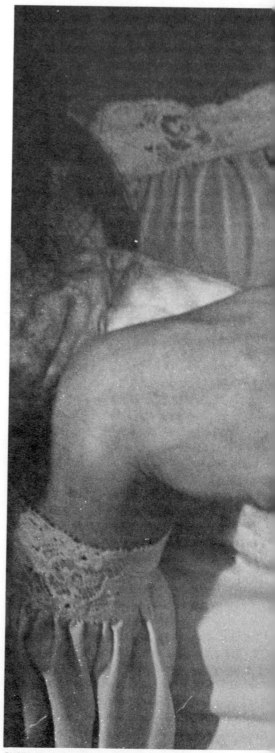

PHOTO BY JOHN BLAIR MITCHELL

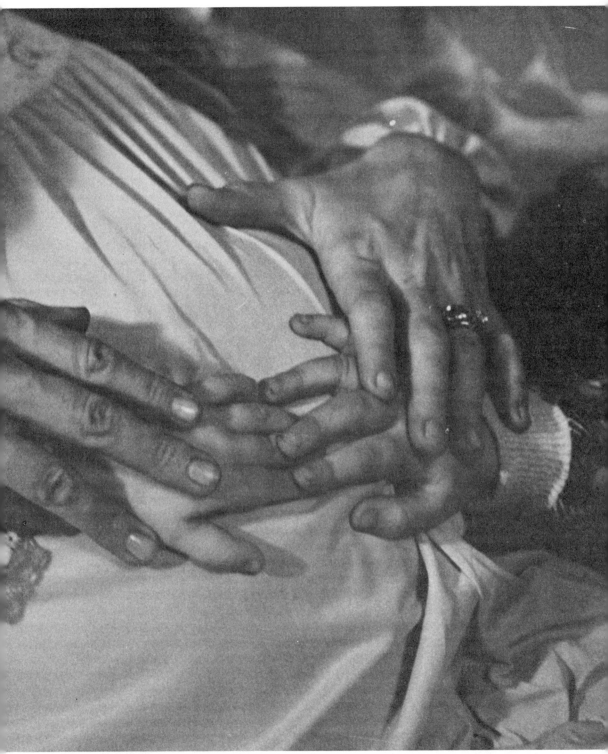

The mother and other family members express their love for the unborn infant, an especially important event since as early as five months after conception a baby develops a consciousness and may even sense whether it is loved or not; unless this love is present, neurosis could have prenatal origins.

out sustained respiration—a total of 200,000 annually in the United States. Dr. Levkoff warned that the newborn babies with this problem who seem to recover may have diminished mental and neurological potential due to brain damage by anoxia.

Dr. Robert O. Bauer, a member of a UCLA research team, reported to the California Medical Association's annual scientific session that many practicing physicians erroneously believe that certain local anesthetics used on the mother as a nerve block do not pass on to the baby. Dr. Bauer has shown that certain widely used anesthetics do indeed pass through the placenta into the fetus.

Normal birth is the most important ingredient for a normal child. Conditions in a home delivery are such that there are few times when the degree of fetal distress warrants a forcep delivery. Because the woman is relaxed in her environment and is mobile and unmedicated, she is able to cooperate during expulsion and push her baby out naturally and unhurriedly into the world. After a patient reexperienced in Primal Therapy his forcep delivery at birth, he concluded this was why he had spent his life waiting to have things done for him. The forceps in this case taught the child from the very beginning that he would not be able to do things by himself.

Delayed deliveries cause untold damage. It is sad to hear that women must be kept panting and blowing, and babies kept from being pushed out, by a doctor's tardy arrival. Harris Sherline, president of United Cerebral Palsy in 1970, publicly warned of this being a cause of palsied and/or retarded babies. With this information, how can nurses still hold a woman's legs together or hold the baby's head back from being born for periods as long as 40 minutes? I have many patients who have relived this particularly frustrating and uncomfortable birth experience. Their subsequent insights all confirm that this delaying practice has disastrous emotional consequences even though the child may be physically normal. One patient reported lifelong feelings of claustrophobia coupled with a feeling of despair that she would inevitably fail if she tried to assert herself. This fundamentally affected her whole attitude toward achievement in life. Through a Primal she connected it to being restrained at birth by a doctor's hand held over her mother's vagina. Many others have reported similar feelings.

One has only to observe a newborn to recognize his helplessness and his dependency on his mother at this time. As the baby is still in a state of exterogestation, the continued period of gestation outside the womb, it has a great need for total care. Birth is too often regarded as the time when a child begins his independence. This is symbolized, so some believe, by the severing of the umbilical cord. But in effect, birth signifies only that the infant is now ready to make a gradual adjustment to his postnatal existence.

The natural rhythm of the childbirth experience is forfeited by introducing drugs or breaking the membranes in order to induce or speed up labor or by performing a Caesarean section. These procedures inflict imprints on the child for the rest of his life. Being born naturally, at the proper time, is an infant's developmental need, and when that need is deprived or hindered, profound and permanent changes can occur. There need not be, however, one overwhelmingly traumatic event in order to permanently affect the child. Tensions can be laid down by a series of small incidents: mismanagement, insensitivity, or inappropriate response—incidents that would least likely occur in the home environment where only one birth is occuring and where much effort will probably be concentrated on the new family member and his comfort.

No longer rocked or lulled in the womb's amniotic fluid, the baby, if not handled securely and gently, is alarmed by the sudden fear of falling. When a baby is first placed on its back, its arms tense and fly outward while it cries frantically. A baby probably feels the same frenzy when held by the feet, upside down, with no support for its body. Some physicians are now finding out that they can fondle and touch or massage the baby to stimulate its breathing pattern. The importance of this new practice can be seen in many Primals. One patient, for example, a forty-eight year old woman, relived her experience of being held upside down and spanked at birth by the doctor who delivered her. The doctor had been very rough in his handling and, during the Primal, the doctor's handprint actually appeared on the woman's leg. This early overload of physical pain could not be integrated into the fragile infant's being at the time and thus remained unresolved and unfelt until the Primal almost a half century later. The body remembers experience as well as the mind.

The warm temperature usually maintained in the family bedroom is far more welcoming to the newborn than the air conditioned cold of a hospital delivery room. And the home born baby is almost always immediately held against the mother's warmth, nursed, and cuddled into bed by her side.

The newborn's ears and eyes are very sensitive. All the clackings, new voices, and bright lights, no longer muffled and subdued by the water of the womb, seem shocking. Frederick LeBoyer is a French doctor who describes his revolutionary methods to make the passage from life in the uterus to life outside a smooth episode for the baby in his book *For Birth Without Violence*. He says that a new-

born perceives sounds the same way a fish does, all over the skin surface. The whole body is like one vast ear.

Circumcision is a tactile assault of unparrelled proportions to a boy child. Once a ritual performed largely among Jews and Moslems, circumcision of the male baby has become routine practice in the United States hospitals. This is not true of the American homes. Perhaps because of the inherent philosophies characterizing home birth couples or because such a procedure would have to be actively sought outside of the home sometime after the birth, circumcision is an exception to the majority of home births.

In most texts the advantages are well listed but the disadvantages are not mentioned. Statements are made to imply that it is painless and does not disturb the baby. One text suggests that the mother not be told the exact time of the procedure, because she might be inclined to think of it in terms of cutting, pain, and blood loss. Well, I believe that the mother should think in those terms, and reconsider the operation. There is little blood loss, true enough, but there is cutting and there is pain. And there is psychological injury to the infant. To observe the operation is evidence enough that the baby experiences pain. Such an unnecessary assault upon a helpless infant, entirely dependent upon its elders, is ghastly to behold.

What are the effects of the circumcision experience? It is one that is frequently relived in Primal Therapy. Patients reliving this event would tell you that it was hardly a slight operation or that it was one of great advantage to them. Those patients who have had Primals about their circumcision all report feeling severe pain.

One patient, a homosexual, had a circumcision Primal after which it became evident to him why he had been unable to have sexual relations with a woman. Each time he had tried to enter a woman he had experienced excrutiating pain— the same pain he experienced when he relived the operation. Obviously this is not to say that circumcision invariably leads to homosexuality but merely that the experience on its own, or compounded with earlier or later trauma, can contribute to neurosis.

The world is so huge and strange to the newborn. Try to imagine how big and looming everything appears from its point of view. Think back to an early time in your life when your father seemed enormously tall. After you grew up, however, he was only 5'8". Or do you remember a room that seemed so large to you as a child but that later seemed small? A newborn *does* see, and he *does* hear, and he *does* feel—and he remembers.

Perhaps the singlemost valuable gift the home birth can offer the newborn is immediate and unrestricted access to his mother, the only person he knows, the greatest comfort and security he can know. His life is so inextricably linked to that of his mother that he cannot understand let alone tolerate separation from her. The baby's immature nervous system makes him so helpless and vulnerable that separation from his mother at this time can cause psychological trauma. Sigmund Freud, Wilhelm Reich, and Otto Rank describe this distress as *separation anxiety* and attribute it to the first anxiety of the baby being separated from his mother.

In giving a definition of neurosis, Dr. Arthur Janov writes in *The Primal Scream*, "Neurosis is a disease of feeling. At its core is the suppression of feeling, and its transmutation into a wide range of neurotic behavior." To leave a baby unsupported by its mother's embrace in a strange and seemingly hostile environment is encouraging permanent trauma.

Because this series of violations I have described may prove too painful for the helpless baby, it may have to shut off its feelings at that time in an effort to survive the agony. Conversely, by providing a warm and gentle environment, the parents have the opportunity to ease the baby's passage into its new phase of existence and materially affect its good adjustment and lasting emotional stability.

The mother is responsible for caring for her infant. Her baby is a dependent, needing, feeling human being. I like the word *needing* rather than *demanding* because demanding implies that the baby is insisting on abnormal, excessive claims rather than expressing his instinctual needs necessary for survival. Demand feeding, for example, might appear in a better light to a new mother if she thought of it as being a time when the baby makes known needs that are established according to his inner law and which must be satisfied if he is to live and grow according to his body's potential. When a baby cries out because he is hungry, he needs to be fed right then. If he is not, then he will learn that his needs will not be met when he expresses them. He will shut off pain. This does not mean that the hunger will go away. It will be suppressed, and a substitute avenue for gratification must be found. For the baby it might be lulling himself by rocking his body or sucking on a finger or a blanket. The unmet need, if unexpressed, will continue through adulthood and take on other symbolic guises like smoking or nail biting.

Margaret Ribble in *The Rights of Infants* says that a baby's mental development will largely depend on how its mother responds to its needs during the first crucial moments of life. Some psychologists refer to this period as one when the parent has to give unconditional love. That suggests that the parent has to be able to give without expecting to receive in return. In order to do that a mother would have to have had all of *her* childhood needs met. Dr. Janov states, "The major reason that I have found that children become neurotic is that their own parents are too busy struggling with unmet infantile needs of their own. The child who suffers the most is the one with the parent who needs the most." This is how neurosis is perpetuated generation after generation.

Ideally, parents should be feeling people. Emotionally disturbed parents are as infectious to their infant as tuberculosis and any adverse contact that they have with their child will be lastingly damaging. It is hoped that when the baby is in the womb he is well-nourished, that there will be no cigarette contamination, no medication, as little DDT infiltration as possible, that he will not hear fearful sounds like screaming from the outside world, and that he will experience a relaxed, tension-free mother. It is further hoped that the mother will be able to help facilitate a normal, smooth birth for her baby because traumatic birth can only cause trauma.

Birth is a normal, natural process. If a birth is normal, there should be no outside intervention. If the birth is not normal, and there has to be intervention, those people who come in contact with this child must help to reassure the child that it is safe, that the trauma it has experienced was trauma of the moment and that now it will be safe. The baby should be soothed and touched and shown every possible consideration. It is admittedly unrealistic to suggest that every child should be born at home, but I feel strongly that every child has a right to be born in as home-like an environment as possible.

I was inspired by a film I saw of Dr. Joseph F. Griggs, a Claremont, California, physician as he participated in a home delivery. His film convinced me of the validity of the home birth experience. It is my contention that a woman and thus her baby are best off under the conditions that are comfortable for her. I began to speak out and tell women of the home birth alternative. Many people responded to this idea and urged me to teach a class designed specifically to meet the needs of home birth couples. Those who attended were surprisingly different in lifestyle, ranging from hippies to very conservative suburbanites. The majority of them had very positive home experiences and now only think of birth in terms of the home. Families who had had previous children in the hospital were particularly vocal. And, of all the resulting babies, no newborn seemed to have had any of the unfavorable practices inflicted upon him that I have written about.

What many hospital personnel seem to consider progress is consolidated care in ever larger centers with more complex machinery. True progress would be the provision for individualized caring and a deeper understanding of the social environment that a laboring woman moves in and how that affects the newborn. Supervised home birth offers the greatest potential for the supportive atmosphere that is necessary for the family unit to consciously participate in a celebration of life that will protect the newborn's emotional needs. Home births already automatically provide personal attention, detailed observation, and constant support within the natural context of the family. Home births can also provide physiological, psychological, and sociological harmony necessary not only to save infants' lives but their sanity as well.

part 3

The Sociological Dimension

By Lester R. Hazell

A Sociological Survey

Home birth is not a phenomenon of poverty and ignorance, but rather one of conviction that there is a better way to have a baby than that prescribed by the prevailing view in today's society. In this, home birth is similar to its philosophic predecessor, the natural childbirth movement. The natural childbirth movement has made significant changes in some aspects of medical practice, and so, too, may the home birth movement if it persists and spreads.

This essay, which is based on research done between 1969 and 1974, examines beliefs and practices relevant to birth among 300 couples who chose to have their babies at home.* All the couples are from the San Francisco Bay Area, and they were known to me because I had helped the couples deliver their children, taught them childbirth preparation classes, or worked with the midwives present at the births. My role as a contributor of expertise involved me in many more of these private situations than if I had been either a simple observer, or even a willing but inexpert participant. All 300 couples responded to a written survey of their views and practices, and this data base was supplemented by indepth interviews with the fathers and mothers of ten home birth families. While my investigation was confined to one geographic area, it is reasonable to expect that similar research in other areas of the United States might yield similar data. For example, the home birth families described later in this book—all from the

---

*This entire research study, entitled "Ethnography of Home Birth in the San Francisco Bay Area," is available for purchase from: ICEA Supplies Center, 1414 Northwest 85th Street, Seattle, Wash. 98117.

Washington, D.C. area—appear to have very similar profiles.

How Are Home Birth Couples Different?

First of all, these couples elected to have their babies at home, with or without medical assistance. The crucial decision was to select home birth; second to that was looking for medical assistance for the delivery. In some instances medical assistance was available; in some it was not or was not sought. This decision to have a home birth with the consideration of medical assistance as secondary was the primary phenomenon that set these people apart from other expectant couples in the San Francisco Bay Area. For whatever reason, it is a safe assumption that for most San Franciscans the presence of a doctor in a hospital is thought to be the essence of having a satisfactory delivery. For the home birth set, however, being at home in familiar surroundings with loved friends was the essential goal.

The typical home birther has graduated from high school, has had some college education, lives in a single family dwelling, has a television set, drives a car and otherwise presents the same outward appearance as any other stereotypic San Francisco Bay area resident. His attitude profile, however, differs from his fellow residents.

The couple favors home birth, and this alone sets it aside. It does not fear potential damaging physical consequences of birth at home, but rather expresses the idea that hospital birth has disadvantages from a psychological standpoint and also can cause unnecessary physical trauma in the name of prevention of pain. Labor is hard work, but not to be feared, and most couples find labor a peak experience. Economically, the home birth couple does not feel particularly secure even though from outward appearances

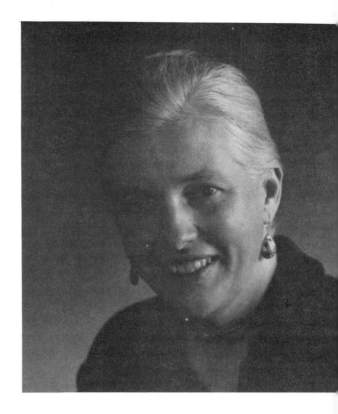

Lester D. Hazell is the author of the best-selling book Commonsense Childbirth, *one of the most comprehensive and readable introductions to "natural" childbirth practices ever written. She holds her M.A. in Psychological/Medical Anthropology from California State University, Hayward, and works as a counselor for Community Mental Health Services in San Francisco. She is a past president of the International Childbirth Education Association and is presently a member of the Board of Directors of that organization. Mrs. Hazell is the mother of two children and lives with her husband in San Anselmo, California.*

it belongs in the same economic strata as other more-or-less middle-income people. The home birth couple emphasizes the importance of good nutrition for mental and physical health and has made something of a study of nutrition. The home birth couple verbalizes an acceptance of death as being not a horror but a part of life. Episiotomy is anathema to the home birth couple and usually represents an unnecessary trauma inherent in hospital birth; for them the responsibility for the outcome of birth is theirs and does not lie in the province of the hospital. Home birth couples spend their leisure time at home or in family-centered pursuits. They do not regard the pain of labor as significant but rather emphasize the transcendental experience as being important. The home birth couple makes no particularly distinctive comments on the topic of sexual intercourse; however, it has very clear ideas on the positive values of bringing children into the world. It doesn't relate to its friends via cocktail parties or coffee clatches. The home birth group is divided on the subject of circumcision, with about four out of five being opposed to the practice. The mother who has had her baby at home breast feeds him enthusiastically with the support of her husband. Most home birth people express deep anger at the medical profession for what they feel is usurpation of the management of normal labor, and they feel the father should be allowed to deliver his baby if he so desires, and most do.

Social Characteristics

One of the characteristics of this group is a hard-to-define level of self-awareness which manifests itself in concern for proper nutrition and a kitchen stocked with health foods, personal libraries dealing with religious topics, philosophy, health, and humanistic psychology.

Another investigator has defined the population interested in natural childbirth, home birth, and breast feeding as part of the "back-to-nature ethos," also noting that they were concerned with ecology and the survival of mankind as a whole. In the years since this investigator's work in 1965, it has been my observation that natural childbirth, breast feeding, and ecological concern have been adopted much more into the wider cultural ethos, while home birth remains by and large culturally unacceptable. The apparently increasing numbers of home births may signal a change in those attitudes.

As is typical of other activities in American society, home birth as observed here was a nuclear family event. Those present were peers, or the children of participants, and not grandparents of the newborn.

Approximately one tenth of the home birth couples studied were not typically middle American. Most of these would be classified as "hip," meaning that they were in a state of rebellion over wider aspects of their lives than was characteristic of the rest of the sample. This group tended to use marijuana, some peyote, and to a lesser degree, LSD. The couples were usually not married but living together in relationships that were not expected to last. They tended to dip for short periods of time into various Eastern religions and to eat limited diets such as the macrobiotic.

In all my experiences with home birth couples in the San Francisco Bay Area, I never found a situation where both partners came from an ethnic minority. Very rarely one member of the couple would be Oriental, but typically the other would be white. Black people are beginning to be found in childbirth classes, but they are upwardly mobile and tend to opt for the "best" physician and hospital available. This tends to mean that they have the usual American birth, leaving responsibility for management to doctors, nurses and other hospital personnel. The lower economic groups are by and large availing themselves of Medi-Cal or county hospital clinics and thereby opting for hospital births in which they, too, leave their decision to the medical profession.

About three quarters of the total home birth group were having first babies. The rest were mostly second births, the first child having been born in the hospital. However, there were also a few families having second and third home births, and one that had had five home births out of six, the first child having been born in the hospital.

Over the time span of the study, 1969 to 1974, there were some changes in attitude. Early in the study the people that were most visible were members of the "hip" community who tended to give the appearance of flaunting the fact that they had had a home birth in the face of all sorts of objections from their parents. As time went on, more and more typical middle class Americans came forward, many of whom had had home births but had revealed their experience only to close friends. With the publication of books like this one, we may find that more and more couples will not only select the home birth alternative, but also be more inclined to share their experience with others.

Helen and Ray Stone

Helen, a native of Wales, was the fifth of six children. Her mother had her first four children at home; Helen was born in the hospital. During a vacation in the United States, Helen met Ray, now the Director of Tours for the Air Force Band. Before they saw each other again, they were engaged by letter. Helen delayed moving until after her graduation from the University of South Wales in Cardiff, where she earned a degree in biochemistry equivalent to the first year of study toward an American Ph.D. The Stones were married eight years ago in the Mormon Temple in Oakland, Calif. They live in Kensington, Md. with their five children. Seven-year-old Raymond was born in a hospital with medication. Samantha, 5½, and Alexandra, 4½, were also born in the hospital, but with natural childbirth. Before the hospital birth of James, now 23 months, Helen, 30, and Ray, 44, studied prepared childbirth. Susana was born four weeks ago at home.

Profiles of Home Birth Families

HELEN: Our first three children were born in military hospitals. I had terrible experiences in them. I had no say-so at all. The procedures were very regimented, and everything was so impersonal. No one took the time to explain anything to me. If only I had known then that home birth was possible in the United States, I would never have gone through all I did.

With my first baby, Raymond, I was in a labor ward. If that's not a frightening experience, I don't know what is, to lie there and to hear everybody else screaming. No one was with me whom I could feel close to, and to hear all the other women around me was horrible. Ray and I had only been married a year.

INTERVIEWS
BY CHARLOTTE WARD

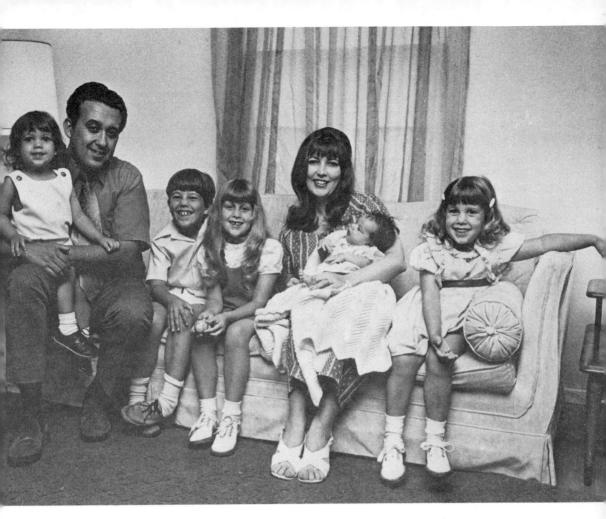

Before that my mother had always been there to help me with everything. If there were ever a time in my life when I needed my husband, it was right then! But in that situation, I was all alone.

Raymond's birth was made *more* difficult by the strained surroundings. The nurse even remarked to me during that time, "Oh, you're not feeling bad enough yet"! They gave me Demerol, then a paracervical block, and finally a low spinal, or "saddle block." I still worry about how those medications affected our first child.

It's been seven years, but I still remember it vividly. I could not even *think* about having more children right away. My husband and I believe in taking our babies as they come, but, at that point, I simply

didn't want to undergo the birth process soon again. I tried to block it out of my mind. That's significant to me. I wouldn't want anyone else to have to go through such distress.

How ironic it is that people go on so about the "safe" hospital births! While I was in the labor room before Samantha was born, my contractions suddenly changed in character. I called the nurse, who came in briefly, laid her hand on my stomach, and told me, "They're just getting harder." Five minutes later I rang again and insisted on her checking. She returned with an intern. He looked in at me from the door and told her, "Oh, give her some Demerol," without even asking me! Almost as an after-thought, he picked up the sheets and suddenly

92

realized that the delivery was imminent. You ought to have seen them scurry to get me to the delivery room and get their masks on. All the time he kept saying to me, "Don't push! Don't push!" As soon as they put me onto the delivery room table, Samantha was born. She came so fast they didn't even have time to put my legs in the stirrups, and I never did push.

During my pregnancy with James, Ray agreed to go with me to Lamaze classes, and we practiced the training exercises at home. This time he was with me in the labor room. The nurse assigned to us had been a midwife in West Virginia, and I had told her that I would have liked to have this baby at home. Perhaps she didn't anticipate how rapidly I was progressing, but I rather think she let me stay in the labor room on purpose. Anyway, moments before Jamie was born, she grabbed a doctor going on duty who just happened to be walking by in the hall. The doctor wasn't scrubbed, of course. She hadn't even washed her hands. The nurse did most of the delivery. She eased the baby's head out, and I didn't even tear. Perhaps Lamaze had a lot to do with that too. So Jamie was born in the labor room. I was glad in many ways, but at the same time, I thought how ridiculous it is to say how safe and *sterile* the hospital delivery is. That labor room wasn't nearly as clean as my bedroom at home. There's no way of knowing who had been there before me or what pathogens were present.

RAY: Everything is wrong about hospitals for having normal babies. Just when a woman should be still and relaxed, she has to move and drive to the hospital. That's not right. Then she goes to a desk and talks to a bunch of strangers to register. The positions she is asked to assume are all wrong—against gravity.

There's just no reason for any of this. The hospital takes over and assumes the upper hand. The mother and father are left out. The baby is brought to them when the hospital wants it and not when the mother and baby, and *father*, need it. Feeding glucose is universal, and we don't think that's right either. Any other sugar than lactose establishes a basic, rather than an acidic, flora in the baby's stomach. This makes him vulnerable to gastro-intestinal disease organisms. The baby needs nursing and wants its mother. It doesn't need a bottle of sugar water.

HELEN: Childbirth is a very sensitive time for me; I am preparing to take care of this tiny, fragile person coming into the world, completely dependent on me and on her father. So, I want to be treated gently, not like an object. In the hospital I never got the feeling that anybody except Ray was concerned about me. The way they scrub at you and get you ready—as though you have no feelings whatsoever. Everything went just as smoothly at home without all that prepping. In the hospital they made me feel afraid I was going to contaminate my own baby. I wish they had treated the birth process as what it is: a fact of life, not a disease.

We felt Susana's birth at home was, in one word, NATURAL. At home we could communicate with the doctor and the nurse because they believe the same way we do. And our family didn't come up against tension-causing situations, which, I believe, precipitate many physical ills. I think that one of the most important needs to be provided for in childbirth is relief from all this tension that so often accompanies births in subtle and unsubtle ways in the hospital. I hemorrhaged after the births of the second, third, and fourth children, and I expected to after Susana. But her birth was so different. With the relaxed atmosphere of having the baby at home and being able to nurse her immediately and at will, I didn't have any trouble at all.

I was so happy with the whole situation. It really wasn't a hard labor, although it was a long one. It was really very easy. And from the first day I could help with the work at home instead of lying in the hospital worrying about how my family was adjusting. The children, of course, were ecstatic, since they could come in and see Momma and the baby at any time they wanted to. And I have *felt* so much better after Susana's birth than after any of the others. I enjoyed going to a ballet at the Kennedy Center a week after she was born!

Ray managed so beautifully looking after the children. They were secure with us all together at home. At a time when our two-year-old might have felt confused and neglected, he had no problems with jealously or loneliness. With past deliveries, this business of Ray's running to and from the hospital had been difficult for everyone. The baby and I wanted to see him, and the children needed him at home.

We sought a home delivery as a part of our attempt to approach life in a more natural way. We are health-food-minded. I enjoyed staying home and eating well right away. When you need nourishing food, you can get exactly what you want in your own kitchen. None of that synthetic hospital fare!

We enjoy a close-knit family, and that led us to think there must be a more natural way of birth. We couldn't see any real advantage to hospital deliveries, and we thought the hospital separation of mother and child was artificial, unnecessary, and actually harmful. I just don't think that most people realize how much the mother and baby need each other right after birth. From the first day Susana expressed her desire to be touching me. She would cry if I put her into the cradle beside my bed, whereas if I just kept her in bed beside me, even when I wasn't holding or nursing her, she would be calm.

Now Ray is as enthusiastic about home births as I am. I have also noticed a difference in him with the babies. He has had a lot more to do with the last two in the infant stage. And he seems a lot more baby-oriented. It was a good feeling having Ray here looking after me during the birth. It meant an increase of love between us. I gained a greater understanding of my husband. We have a good, close marriage relationship anyway. Sharing this birth was an added bonus. Having Susana at home was a good, solidifying experience.

Nancy and Wally Knapp

NANCY: When I got pregnant with Christopher, I didn't even know the term *Lamaze*. I just knew that whatever I had seen as far as childbirth in nursing school was what I was *not* going to do. There was no dignity in that. Maybe another factor was that I was not willing to surrender my control to someone else. I did know about Grantly Dick-Read.

Then when we talked to an obstetri-

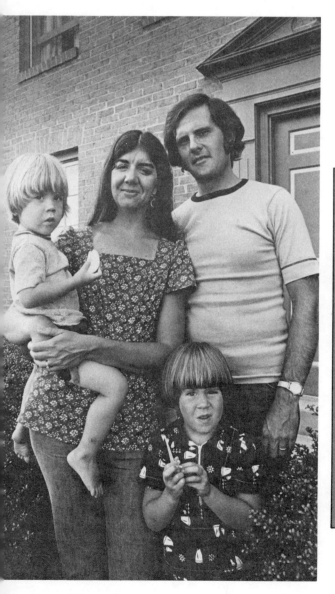

Nancy, 31, and Wally, 33, live in Potomac, Md. Wally is the Director of Computer Systems Development at American University in Washington, D.C., and Nancy is a Registered Nurse, now working as an assistant to Dr. Brew and completing her B.A. in Nursing at American University. The Knapps have two children. Christopher, 5, was born in Georgetown University Hospital by prepared childbirth and no medication. Jeremy, 2½, was born at home. Wally and Nancy took the Childbirth Education Association's series of six childbirth classes and Nancy joined La Leche League in preparation for Christopher's birth. During this learning period, Nancy became so interested in "supported childbirth," that she became qualified to teach for C.E.A. and do labor support, first in the hospital and then in the home, assisting Dr. James Brew.

95

cian, he said about labor procedure, "Whatever you want to do," but it became painfully obvious to me that what *that* meant was whatever I wanted to do only included what he wanted me to do. The day I broached the subject of husbands in the delivery room, he leaned back in his chair behind his desk and assumed a very fatherly manner. "Now, Mrs. Knapp," he told me, "You don't want to do that because we know about Semmelweis and childbed fever. We know about infections if you've got someone else in the delivery room." I just said to him, "I'm sorry. I know enough about asepsis to know that's not valid. We obviously are not together on this." By mutual agreement, we severed our relationship and I looked for someone else.

WALLY: He was a typical father image—a nice little old man who said, "Now don't you worry, Sweetie, I'm just going to take you through this terrifying experience and I'm just going to bring this baby right into the world for you." It was obvious that he wasn't the answer for us. I feel sad about all the women who get frightened in a situation like that but don't have the courage to say that isn't the answer, there has to be a better way. Many couples will continue in a bad situation rather than take responsibility themselves and make a decision to change doctors. I'm awfully glad we did.

NANCY: At that same time I was getting involved with the League and C.E.A. I began to realize that if I had any hopes of doing anything with prepared childbirth, I was really in the wrong place with that kind of doctor. We sought out a supportive doctor, and Dr. Brew came highly recommended. He delivered Christopher and Wally was with me as my coach.

WALLY: Back in those days (1969), there still weren't that many natural deliveries at Georgetown. There were nurses that had still never seen one and doctors who had never delivered one. We had quite an entourage back in the student section. Back then, a woman wasn't supposed to stand up right after delivery. Nancy got up immediately and walked down the hall. The nurses tried to get her back in bed.

NANCY: They came dashing after me saying, "You're not supposed to get up yet!" We delivered at 7:30 one night and came home with Christopher the next morning at 11 o'clock. I had to observe the 12-hour nursery rule. I couldn't get around it at that time. That was a real difficulty for me. I got to nurse him after he was born before he went to the nursery, and then Wally and I went back to the postpartum room. I slept for about an hour and then I walked back and forth to the nursery, probably 12 times that night. I just couldn't sleep. I was very excited, very elated, and I very much felt lost that here *I* was with a new baby and there *he* was down the hall. My one consolation is that, as far as I know, he slept that entire time. Every time I went down to the nursery, he was asleep. I was able to talk them out of the last two hours because we were going home. That was all a frustration to me. I decided that I was not going to go through that again. I was not going to be in a situation where I had a new baby and I couldn't just curl up with it and nurse it.

WALLY: I think the assumption of most medical people is that when you have a baby, you're sick. Only sick people are in the hospital, so the baby must be sick. Therefore, the baby must spend 12 hours in the nursery. The cold

96

fact is that most babies are born well. If a woman's had a baby she's well, too. So why go to the hospital and observe its rules? There's nothing abnormal about having a child. There's nothing that requires the concept of sickness. There's no association. I think that we've inherited a lot of conditioning and there have been attempts to justify this. I think that's what's sick.

It was very easy for us to make the decision to have a home delivery.

NANCY: Yes, I think we always knew. We had talked about it with the first one, just briefly, and decided that it wasn't for us the first time. After our experience at the hospital, we just knew. It's not that it was so negative, there was just nothing to it.

WALLY: I think the hospital is very mechanical and technological, especially when it is very unnecessary. Nancy and I talked at some length about the risk involved in a home birth, but it didn't worry me. The decision finally came down to mundane considerations like, "It's a nuisance to drive all the way downtown," and I could see no justification for spending over $300. It was easy to do it here. We had a really good nurse who was to be present, and we had complete faith that Dr. Brew had made a good judgment in agreeing to it. There weren't any distraught moments. It just seemed like the natural way to do it. People have been having babies at home for centuries. Since the mortality rate is not improving in this country, with all the hospital care, hospitals just don't seem to be the total answer. It just wasn't a big deal for me. I will say that it didn't hurt to have a wife who is a nurse.

NANCY: The whole experience of having a baby at home is phenomenal. There

was an emotional preparation I had to make, realizing there was some slight risk involved. I had to deal with that risk. Maybe that's because of my medical upbringing. Anyway, for me there are far more risks in delivering in hospitals— from the standpoint of errors and infections—than there are in delivering at home. I would say, too, that the ease with which the whole process took place certainly facilitated our incorporating a second child into our family. From the emotional standpoint, we wanted to be able to have the new baby with us and we didn't want to leave Christopher. He was 2½ when Jeremy was born. I was not prepared to go off and leave him and I wasn't prepared to present him with a new baby coming back from the hospital. While we had the baby, Christopher was here in the house, playing with our friend, Jean.

WALLY: We didn't have that consideration with the first birth. We just closed up the house and went downtown. But with the second child, there's a lot more planning to do—getting everything to jell so that it works out well. It's very easy to have the second child at home, because you don't have to make a lot about nothing. The birth was certainly no trauma for Christopher.

NANCY: It was so rapid. I found it a little harder to cope with than the first one, where I was able to document the separate phases as they came. Jeremy's labor was a lot of contractions all piled together—all happening very, very fast. The morning I decided I was in good labor, as opposed to Braxton-Hicks contractions, I went to see Dr. Brew. Wally and I sat in his office for an hour, but he didn't come in. Since I had no contractions there, we decided to come back home. Wally went on to work and I took

97

a warm bath and went to bed. I called Wally back about noon, Jan got here about 1 o'clock, and the baby was born at 2:45.

WALLY: It's very difficult for me to have much empathy for women who assume that childbirth is a very painful process, because I have participated in two births and it wasn't that way. It's kind of hard for me to relate to people who grow up with old wives' tales and cling to them without opening their minds to new possibilities.

NANCY: What's funny is that Dr. Brew didn't make it to my own home delivery. When we came to the realization that he was on his way but wasn't going to be there, Jan said, "What do you want to do?" And I said, "What do you mean, 'What do I want to do? I want to *deliver!*'" He arrived about half an hour after Jeremy, in time to check the baby and have some champagne.

What I liked best was the ease with which the event took place. It just fitted into our lives. Jeremy was born mid-afternoon. We enjoyed "exploring" the baby, sharing and talking about him together; friends brought us dinner; we settled Christopher for the night; and Wally and I—and Jeremy—went to bed at 7 o'clock! I really got a good night's sleep, except for waking up to nurse the baby. It was all so restful, so peaceful!

There's no comparison with my experience in the hospital, where I spent all night going back and forth to the nursery. Every time I passed the nurses' station, I got another glass of orange juice because there was nothing else to eat. There was *no* food available after I delivered, and I was starving. I kept thinking, "My blood sugar's really down, I'm tired, and I'm going to be in bad shape." So, I kept getting milk and orange juice all night.

WALLY: People don't have to be treated like machines, like they don't have feelings. There's nothing more drab than a labor room. Those rooms don't even have pictures on the walls. They're like being in a prison cell, and a woman can be in one for long hours. Then there are rules, such as you can't have food and drink during labor. One thing that bothered me a lot with Christopher's birth was their moving Nancy from the labor room to the delivery room. It was really hard on her, I know that for a fact. It's all very structured. Things they thought of 50 years ago, they still cling to—for everybody. It wasn't justifiable then and it's still not.

The medical profession is reacting to the mortality rate with more instruments, like fetal monitors of the heart, the amniotic fluid, and so on. The fact of the matter is that these things are not going to make much difference. They're hooking these normal babies up to all these electronic gadgets—trying to solve human problems with technology even where it doesn't relate. The percentage of children who are born without complications is fantastically high—96–98 percent. They burden the vast majority with the problems of a small minority. That seems like over-reaction to me.

NANCY: That's why we appreciate Dr. Brew so much. He has been able to determine that fine line between practicing "dynamic" obstetrics, as he calls it, where the obstetrician interferes too much, and just letting labor take its own course without any assistance. He's a rare person. I just can't understand why many doctors don't recognize that and use similiar foresight in their own practices. Home births are so satisfying all the way around.

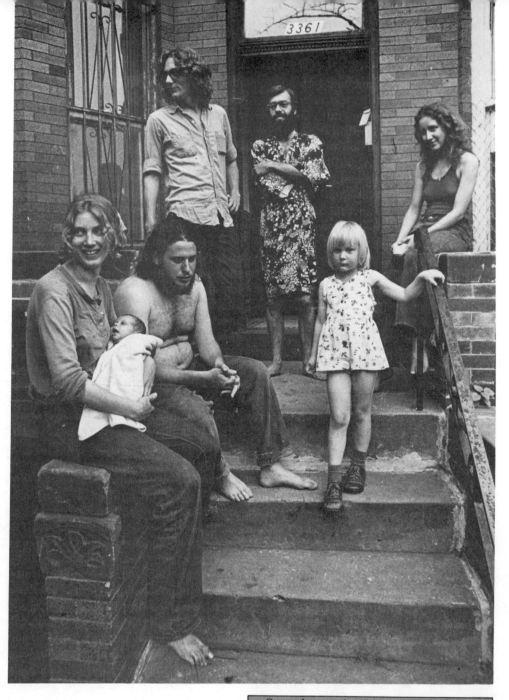

Severine Campbell
and Lenny Moss

Severine and Lenny (left front) live among their friends in a commune in Washington, D.C. Janet Epstein attended the birth of their first child, 2½-week-old Juche, a name that means "self-reliance" in Korean. While Lenny, 21, takes care of the baby, Severine, 21 works at the Community Bookshop in Washington.

SEVERINE: My first consideration was having the baby at home. I really didn't look into the hospitals. I have a real difference of opinion with the hospital system in America. From what I've heard and in talking to women who've had babies and to Phyllis Stein, who taught the Lamaze course, I believe having a child in the hospital would prove a very alienating experience. Even if you go through natural childbirth, there is a lack of continuity. You are removed from the home and put into special sterilized surroundings that don't have a lot to do with your own life. People I'm close to who have had babies in the past five or six years have felt they were being over-controlled in the hospital; they were even frightened at what was happening to them. I just didn't want to go through that.

LENNY: I feel very connected to the idea of home birth. Being in control of the situation, having some self-determination about the process and not being funneled into an institution is very important. We never thought much about a hospital. Birth is a natural process which does not need to be mystified as it is in the present system. Natural childbirth is a de-mystifying process as far as the natural functions of the human body. The idea of a child being born in a hospital and then left alone in a nursery is repulsive. Why should a newborn child be subject to a strife kind of environment right after birth?

It was important to have a number of our friends with us at the time of birth and right after. We had been talking to people about our concepts of collective rearing and breaking down the nuclear family orientation. Such a project would be best seen right from the beginning when people could actually experience the birth and be around a few days after.

There's a good feeling about how you can relate to the child and share a child-rearing experience. We spoke to many people and they were interested in being there. There'd have been more people present if it hadn't been such a short labor and everything hadn't happened so quickly.

SEVERINE: Dr. Brew came about a half hour after Juche was born. He had not planned to come for the birth. We just asked for Janet to be here. I really enjoyed the experience of just having a woman deliver the baby. It somehow made it more intimate to me.

Lenny and I and another woman whom I work with came to class with me because I had wanted her to be present at the birth. Nobody made it—well, hardly—because it was so short. I was only in labor for about five hours. Janet came just as Juche was ready to be born. Ralph and a woman named Jean, and Natalie made it just before the baby was born. And Suzanne made it just after. Somebody had to go wake her up. It seemed so much easier than I had expected. It was a little bit hard not having anyone around who really knew what was happening. Lenny was with me. Things went so fast. I had read all the right books, but I didn't follow any of the right patterns. I didn't realize I was going that fast. I kept waiting for things to get worse. I was really glad when Janet showed up so that she could tell me what was happening. She came maybe half an hour before the birth. I was very relieved.

LENNY: Before Janet came, I got to feeling a little unnerved. I picked up *Our Bodies, Ourselves* to read the emergency procedures, but I wasn't absorbing very much. I wasn't in the best frame of mind for reading.

100

SEVERINE: The birth was very uncomplicated. There just didn't seem to be any complications or difficulties. During my pregnancy I did appreciate Dr. Brew's attitude. He didn't assume that I was going to have the baby in the hospital. He asked me how I wanted to have the baby. I felt reassured. I didn't have a lot of questions about the actual delivery. He had such a matter of fact attitude—it just seemed like such a simple thing.

By the time the doctor came, I was ready for a shower. Word had gotten out and the people who had planned to be there came by and spent the rest of the day with me. It was like a celebration in many ways. We had a big breakfast —bagels, cream cheese, and champagne. Everyone took days off work to share this time with us.

The really important thing was that there was no separation. I had Juche with me. I didn't feel harassed by people around me. I didn't have to deal with interns or nurses, didn't have to ask for anything. Just very simple. I think it's important to the child to have that initial contact.

Juche was very alert. She was born with her eyes open, kicking and screaming. I have nothing to compare it with except stories of hospitals from other women. It's really important not to have an alienating experience—really important to have a natural experience, an organic experience that I will remember for the rest of my life. I'm very much against the use of drugs unless it's absolutely necessary. I've heard that with spinal blocks and such things there can be long-term back problems. I've read a lot of studies that drugs can cross the placenta and have some effect on the early development of the child. Juche was very alert when she was born and very conscious, so I think that not taking drugs made a great deal of difference. There is an over dependence on a lot of drugs during childbirth. I suspect that people just don't know what is happening to them, so they're afraid. I feel very strongly about the fact that women aren't told what is happening to them. My sister and close friends didn't know where to seek the information, so they didn't and remained totally ignorant about their pregnancies and births and the possible effects the drugs could have on the children or them. It's not worth the risk.

Psychologically, for the woman, it's important to have that constant sensation, that constant awareness of being in touch with her body during the whole process of birth. It makes a great deal of difference in her attitudes towards the child and the whole experience. I have fond memories. In retrospect, I don't feel it was that painful, never unbearable. It wouldn't frighten me to go through it again. The initial contact with Juche, *our* initial contact, was very important.

LENNY: Spending the first day in the nursery is just despicable treatment for a new baby. The immediate togetherness between mother and child and others is quite important. Psychologically, emotionally, socially—it's very beneficial to have a home birth. In our situation, not only was I able to be there, but so were our friends as well. This develops a sense of continuity and affection with the child.

101

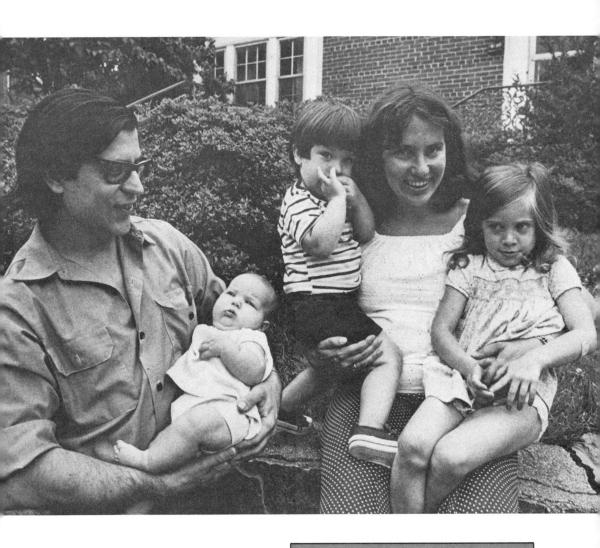

Virginia and Mario Barraco-Marmol

Virginia and Mario reside in Washington, D.C., with their three children. Maria, 4, and her brother, Ruy, 2½, were born in the hospital with natural childbirth. Their new baby sister, Consuelo, 2 months, was born at home, attended by Dr. James Brew and Janet Epstein. Editor of the Organization of American States *Chronicle*, Mario, 41, came from Argentina eight years ago. His name, like that of many of his countrymen, reflects his Italian heritage. While dating Mario, Virginia, 31, began to study Spanish in earnest. After their marriage five years ago, she became a free-lance Spanish language translator.

VIRGINIA: I always dreamed of having my baby at home. As a young girl back in Missouri, my attempts to imagine childbirth were fairly down to earth. I had witnessed the birth of a calf one summer in the country. I will never forget how the mother cow patiently and gently licked the half-drowned little calf into a cute furry animal. It was an emotional thrill to watch an inert form slowly come to life before my eyes. That made me want to witness the same miracle in my own child.

Birth is a moment when I feel most vulnerable. I want the person I love at my side to encourage and protect me, to share in a thrilling and joyful experience. I would simply feel incomplete to experience this alone.

My father, who is a doctor, explained clinical aspects of childbirth to me, but this didn't really satisfy me. It was like trying to describe a symphony by explaining how sounds are produced in violins and trumpets. I can remember unspoken information being passed from my mother when we sat together as she nursed my younger brother. I still feel that the most beautiful way for a child to learn about birth and care of a newborn baby is from his own mother and father within the setting of his own home.

In my eighth month of pregancy with Consuelo, I visited the zoo. I was struck by the elaborate precautions taken to avoid intruding on the privacy of all the pregnant animals. There was a roped off enclosure with guards to prevent anyone getting near enough to disturb the pregnant rhinoceros. I noticed even more precautions with the expectant gorilla, for which the whole wing of the building was roped off. Why should I be considered less delicate than these animals? Because they did not have to send to India or Africa for a specimen of me?

When I became pregnant with my first child, I tried to find a doctor who would come to my home. The first doctor I talked to said, "Don't bother your pretty little head with that. Leave it to me." He apparently thought of childbirth in terms of pulling the white rabbit out of the hat. And he, as the magician, could hardly be expected to reveal his trade secrets. And I, as the hat, could hardly be expected to have an opinion. I just decided not to go back to him.

Although I called the medical referral service of the District of Columbia Medical Board, they told me that there were no doctors in the area who would deliver at home. I later found out this was not true. After getting the names of several doctors who would permit natural childbirth, I resigned myself to giving birth in the hospital. I was pleased that at least I did not have to have anesthesia, that I could have my husband with me, and that I could leave soon after the delivery. To prepare, I went to Parent and Child classes.

When my first child was born, Mario was with me at the hospital. Although it was against hospital regulations, the doctor let me nurse the baby right after birth, but he cautioned me to hold her through the sheet and not to touch her with my bare hands! Nursing was just as easy as it had seemed when I watched my mother. It was a very beautiful birth. By contrast, the woman next to me in the recovery room was drugged out of her mind. She didn't even know she'd had a baby. She asked me why I felt so good. I was grateful for the experience I had had. There were some silly restrictions. I was, for instance, ordered to wear a bra at all times, even in bed. When the nurses discovered I did not have one, they sent my friend out to buy one. They threatened me with a breast binder if I did not wear a bra, but they finally gave up. Maria was brought to me wrapped up in what looked like a little straight jacket, and I was ordered not to unwrap her, look at her body, or try to change her. Mario and I couldn't wait to get her home with us, out of the eyes of hospital vigilance.

I was in the same hospital for the birth of our second child Ruy. It was a terrible experience. The nurse came into the labor room and insisted I have Demerol. I was feeling fine, but she took my blood pressure and said it was too high. I panicked and concentrated all my thoughts on lying still and relaxing. A few minutes later, when my back was turned toward the door, the same nurse sneaked up and was about to give me a hypodermic "to make me feel more comfortable." I insisted on talking to my doctor. He had gone off duty and an associate took over. I told him, "My problem is not with my blood pressure. If you would just get rid of the nurses, I'm sure my blood pressure would be fine." After a few minutes of being left alone, he checked again and told me, "Well, well. Mind over matter. It's perfectly normal now. You're six centimeters dilated and the baby will be born within the hour."

I felt it would be sooner, but I didn't want to cause any more trouble. My husband took one look and said, "Don't you think the baby's head is coming now?" I said, "Yes, but I don't want to argue anymore." He ran for the doctor. The nurses rushed in and tried to push the bed into the hall, so that the baby wouldn't be born in the labor room. That's against hospital regulations. Ruy didn't wait. He came shooting out, along with the placenta. The nurses took him to the delivery room, and Mario and my doctor came back surprised to find no baby. They brought him back to me, wrapped hastily in an adult hospital gown, while a meeting was called to decide what to do with him. They couldn't put him with the other babies in the nursery for fear of contaminating them. I nursed him, enjoying the humor of the whole situation. Sadly, they decided to put Ruy in an incubator and isolate him from the others. That evening, when the babies were brought to their mothers, mine was not included. They said it was too soon, that he could not nurse until the next day. "But he already has," I said. Soon I heard him crying, then wailing desperately. He cried until 10:30 and I was told that my blood pressure was high again. I told a sympathetic nurse, "The only thing the matter with me is that I want my baby." Finally I was desperate. What could I do short of walking through the door and seizing him? Half bursting with anger, I opened the door a crack to where the nurse was sitting in a chair by the baby watching him cry and asked how I could get him. The answer from a pediatrician, Russel Bunai, was a merciful order: "To be fed on demand."

Finally my poor little thing was brought to me. I took him with tears in my eyes. His face was red and wet and his whole body was heaving with tears so that he had to slow down his gasps a little bit to be able to nurse. Maybe he recognized my odor, since he had nursed at birth. He quieted down immediately and began to nurse very efficiently and seriously. If that was all he wanted, it seemed such a simple thing to bring him across the hall, but then, I was not used to hospital procedure. The next nurse on duty seemed to understand. She said she would leave him with me as long as I wanted. Needless to say, I did not ring. I just dozed off and on all night, happy to have the warm little body beside me. I vowed that if I ever had another baby, it would not be born in the hospital, no matter how good the hospital was supposed to be.

A year later, I was pregnant with our third child. I began reading all I could find on home birth: Helen Wessel's *Natural Childbirth in the Christian Family;* Doris Haire's pamphlet, *The Cultural Warping of Childbirth;* Lester Hazell's *Common Sense Childbirth.* I practically memorized Gregory White's *Emergency Childbirth.* One day I felt I could do it alone at home and it was so foolish to worry about such a simple thing; the next day I felt I should conquer my distaste for the hospital and submit for the good of the family.

At the last minute, when I was a full eight months pregnant, I found by chance the doctor I had been looking for. I asked the pediatrician, Dr. Bunai, casually what he thought about home births. He surprised me by saying thoughtfully, "I think, given certain conditions, it is perfectly all right." He recommended Dr. James Brew and Janet Epstein.

When I went into labor, I prepared my room. Now that I was faced with total freedom, I couldn't quite decide how to have the baby. Should I draw the curtains and give birth in the serene tranquility of semi-darkness? I couldn't get over the feeling that it was a rather natural event, so I ended up leaving the curtains and windows open to let in the warm air and sunlight and a view of the azaleas and cherry trees blooming in the yard below. When Jan arrived she was wearing an attractive denim pants suit, rather than a white starched uniform and cap. I was grateful to her for not bringing the hospital into the home. She sat down casually at the foot of the bed and was so much fun to talk to I forgot I was in the middle of labor. My husband and our best friends came in to talk, and our two children played outside with a puppy we were keeping for the weekend. Later, they wandered in and out, saw part of the birth and were excited to hold their newborn sister's hand, but the new baby, Consuelo, was hard put to compete with the visiting puppy!

Dr. Brew arrived in a most attractive suit, silk shirt, and tie fastened with a gold tie clip, looking as if he had come straight from church. Later he merely rolled up his sleeves a little and delivered the baby, without getting a single spot on his shirt.

Everyone, Dr. Brew, Janet Epstein, our friends Becky and Dick, and Mario, were all standing at the foot of the bed watching for the baby to appear. It was strange, but in such an exposed position, I did not feel in the least embarrassed, nor did anyone else seem to. The body was for a different purpose now, and its parts had a different meaning. "Here it comes, it's coming!" exclaimed several voices at once, and Mario grabbed the camera. I watched the mirror and first saw the opening enlarge a little, then suddenly a round tight circle of hair, then the whole top of the head appeared. I couldn't keep from exclaiming as the baby's head popped out. Then one firm push and the whole body spiraled out, a kicking, squirming, pink, 9 pound, 10 ounce baby girl!

After the doctor and nurse left, I went downstairs with my husband and friends to the patio. There we all sat, eating pizza and sipping wine, on a warm sunny day under a blossoming cherry tree, I with a new baby on my lap still rosy from birth. I was thoroughly happy. As she nursed, my own love for Consuelo was so strong I think I would have cried from pure emotion if I had not had a physical way to express my love for her. At last, birth had been just as I had imagined it when I was 12. This time I really felt as if I had had my first child.

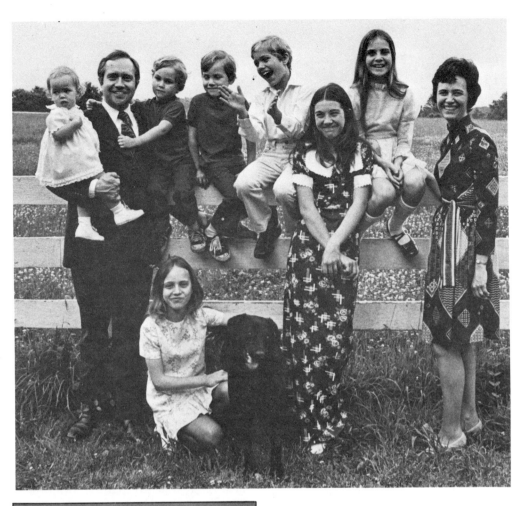

Karen, 37, and Dallas, 38, live in Silver Spring, Md. where Dallas founded Leadership Systems, Incorporated. Principally an executive training center, it can also assist a client in assessing applicants and recommending individuals to fill particular positions within the company's hierarchy. The Merrell family, Mormons by faith, consists of eight children, with another baby born in March, 1975. Fourteen-year-old Ann, 12-year-old Kay, 11-year-old Joan, 9-year-old Paul, and 5-year-old Mark were all born in the hospital with medication. John, 3, and Ilene, 1, were born at home under the care of Dr. Brew and Janet Epstein.

Karen and Dallas Merrell

KAREN: My inspiration for a home birth was an article in a church publication. It said that life has been taken out of the home. Practically the only kind of living that's done there anymore is that people go home to eat, sleep, and change clothes—that's all. We're rarely allowed to die at home, or even to be very sick, or to be born. This idea really made an impression on me. I decided right then that I would like to bring living back into our home. My first five children were born in the hospitals, but that was before I had this realization.

106

I don't believe I ever made a conscious decision to have a baby at home. It just kind of gradually evolved. It was some time later that I found out that Dr. Brew delivered at home. When I asked him if it would be possible, he looked at my record of normal deliveries and said, "I don't see why not."

It really wasn't a question of economics for us, although I am a tight-wad type. I just got to thinking about the kind of non-care I got in the hospital that I paid so much for It really kind of aggravated me when I thought about it. I had always shivered through the whole process. From the time I had entered the hospital till I left, I had been cold. I thought it was a part of childbirth until I had a baby at home and finally just had to fling off the blankets. I suddenly realized that the chill had nothing to do with birth; it was simply that the hospital staff didn't care enough or understand what the needs of women are at that particular time to keep the labor and delivery rooms adequately heated!

I really appreciated having my husband with me at home. He had been in the hospital with me when Mark was born, but he was more an observer than a participant. I was grateful for that, but how much better it was to have him with me and really be able to help me. I had quite a long labor with John, the first born at home. He weighed ten pounds, the largest one we've had, and that took ten hours of labor. Dallas helped support my back during that time. Gosh, I don't know how I'd have gotten through it without him.

Our last born, Ilene, was so much easier. I was glad I had had John first. Although I did always have a paracervical block in the hospital, I found that it isn't much harder to have children naturally. I think we're kind of scared into the idea that we can't do this on our own anymore. I have this other funny quirk. I don't like to be too dependent on society for anything, because I have seen too many instances where society hasn't come through. This prompted me to learn to make my own soap—just to see if I could do it. We buy grain and grind our own flour for the bread I make, and we've learned to can all kinds of fresh produce for the winter. I think if we ever had to be on our own, we'd do all right, and I even think I could have a baby without Dr. Brew now. That gives me a great feeling of independence!

Having these last two babies born at home has made a difference to everyone. As much as fathers may try to intellectualize how bad childbirth is, unless they are there they cannot understand what a woman has gone through. My husband came from a farm and he had a tendency to relate my experience to the animals he grew up with. He has always had a deep respect for life, but he mentions quite often that he has a new, special feeling since the birth of our last two children. Even the one in the hospital that he was present for made a difference. With the others, of course, he was out in the waiting room. I just feel really bad to think what he's missed, but glad that he finally found out. He always used to have a tendency to think that tiny babies were too fragile for him to handle. He's gotten over that feeling now.

It was great for our other children, too. We have what we call "family night," which is something we do every week. We don't even answer the telephone if it rings because there are so few sacred nights left just to be with your family. The Morman church sets aside this night throughout the church that families spend together. This particular one was very close to Ilene's time to be born. We spent the evening talking about each one of the children's births, the special story and circumstances surrounding it, and just how unique each individual is and what great qualities each added to our family by his presence. I had saved some pictures from *Life* magazine showing the child, the fetus in the embryonic fluid, beautiful shots, just fascinating. We talked about the process of birth, how it is the product of love. It was just one of those really special experiences. After Dallas and I had tucked all of the children into bed, we went upstairs to our room and my waters broke. When the children awoke in the morning, there was this new little baby sister. Dallas wrapped the baby up and took her down and put her in our oldest daughter's arms. Ann was asleep, and it was about 5:30 in the morning. She just could not believe it when she woke up and found the baby there.

I hate to think we might have missed this sharing by being in the hospital. We could never duplicate that experience if we tried. It has a special meaning for us.

I found in the hospital I had to fight the nurses to get to nurse my babies. Very often they'd fed the babies first. Then, when it was time for me to get mine, he just didn't want to nurse. It just went so smoothly at home. I had the baby there whenever it needed me and I needed it. People ask me how I get any rest at home. That is no problem. I found in the hospital that a nurse was constantly coming in at 5:30 A.M. when I was still sleeping and waking me. For Ilene's birth, Dallas arranged to take three days off, and a friend who is a nurse watched the baby very closely for the first twenty-four hours. That first night I got a good sleep, except for the nursing periods, and then we just sailed along beautifully.

Birth at home is wonderful. I'm surrounded by the things that mean a lot to me and by the people who mean a lot to me. I never felt strong enough to have a lot of visitors in the hospital, but at home it's fine. Now, when my friends find out I've had a baby, they're over immediately—as if they've got to see for themselves that we're all right. I'm so relaxed, and it's a time to celebrate. I just hope I never have to go back to the hospital—for anything! With this last baby, we had the best insurance coverage. I could have gone to the hospital and stayed for several days without paying a cent, but that's just not what I wanted. You see, I am an extremely modest and private person by nature, and I find home birth a far less public way to have a baby.

ANN: When I woke up and found I was holding a new baby, I thought I was dreaming or maybe Daddy was teasing me. I said, "Are you kidding me?" I really thought it was just a doll. Then the baby cried and I started shaking. I told him to take her back because I might drop her. I was too excited.

We think Ilene is really special. I think our family is closer for having had her at home. Just the night before we'd had that family night, and then there she was the next morning. Ilene's really smart. I don't know whether that has anything to do with her being born at home or not. She's really sweet. I may have my first couple of children at the hospital and then all the others at home, because I think it's better at home. My friends think so, too. They think it's really neat. All of them wish their mothers could have some of their kids at home. When Ilene was born that morning, I called them up. They were all so excited.

It just seems sort of old-fashioned to have a baby at home. Friends came over, mostly from our church, and brought us dinners and visited with my mom. The whole feeling in the house was neat—just really special.

108

Mary and Fortunato Mendes, Jr.

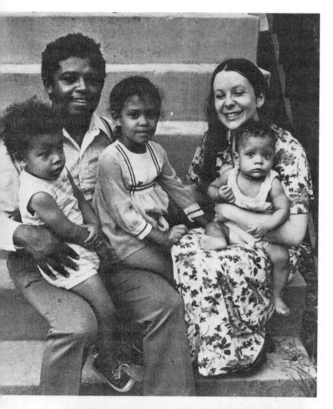

Mary, 27, and Fortunato, 30, moved from Rhode Island eight years ago to study in Washington, D.C. After graduating from Howard University Law School, Fortunato established his own law firm in which he handles both civil and criminal work. Mary ranks second in her senior class at Howard University School of Medicine. After graduation in 1975, she has chosen to do her residency in the field of Obstetrics and Gynecology. Mary and Fortunato have three children. Andrea, who is five years old, had a medicated birth in the hospital. Both of her younger brothers, Fortunato (F.J.) III, 2, and Asante, 8 months, were born at home. They were attended by Dr. Brew and Janet Epstein.

MARY: I had wanted to have natural childbirth with my first child, Andrea. My obstetrician was not cooperative. He suggested an epidural, which I agreed to have. Then, when I got into the hospital, I was in the hardest part of labor, and the nurse said, "Oh, dear, let us put you to sleep. You don't have to go through this." At that point, she sent Fortunato out. Although they had an epidural scheduled, by the time I got into the delivery room, they had changed this to a general anesthesia. When the nurse said, "Gas," I thought she was going to give me a puff, and then I'd be awake the rest of the time. Much to my surprise, she kept the mask on me. It was a suffocating feeling. I wanted to tell them to take it off, but I couldn't say anything because it was over my mouth. When I woke up, I was very happy because I had Andrea, but I was disappointed. I had wanted to see her born.

Soon afterwards I saw my friend Leslie have a home delivery. I enjoyed it. I thought it was fantastic after she had the baby to be lying there in her own bed with her baby in her arms, nursing. It was just such a beautiful way to have a child that I decided I wanted home birth for myself.

I had all kinds of misgivings because people said, "What if there is an emergency?" But Dr. Brew, who was Leslie's doctor, reassured me that he brought along his own resuscitation equipment and his own sterile field, that is, sterile instruments wrapped in sterile cloths. I had read that infants are more susceptible to hospital infections than they are to germs around their own homes, and hospital infections also tend to be resistant to antibiotics. Just in terms of lessening the chances for infection and because I wanted my children to determine their own feeding schedules, I chose home delivery. When I talked to some of the doctors at school, a pediatrician among them, they all said, "Ridiculous! Just absurd, archaic!" Freedmans Hospital, attached to Howard University, doesn't even allow the husband in the *labor* room, to say nothing of the delivery room.

FORTUNATO: Whatever Mary wanted to do, that was fine with me. I felt good about it. I didn't have any qualms. Some of my neighbors back in Rhode Island had home deliveries, mostly by accident. They'd go to the hospital to be checked and then come right back home again. So, the idea of our having a home birth didn't seem extraordinary. I was at the hospital when we had Andrea and had the usual experience. When the baby was born, I saw her before my wife because Mary was still asleep. I was there with the baby when Mary woke up.

MARY: I wanted to have the baby in my own bed. After having the baby, I wanted to be in our own house. I wanted the baby with me all night. I really wanted to have the comfort of home, not the coldness of the hospital. I didn't want the baby kept away and washed and fed by someone else.

While doing my clerkship in obstetrics and gynecology I delivered a few babies at D.C. General Hospital. The doctors over there did a pelvic about every half hour during a woman's labor. That is really unnecessary. The women I saw were mostly between 14 and 18 years old, with no childbirth preparation, and in terrible pain. They were terrified. I tried to explain to them, "Pant like a dog," during a contraction, but they were too scared and couldn't seem to relax with the contractions at all. A lot of the doctors were callous toward the women. They would come out of the labor rooms and say to each other, "Do you really think she's in such pain?" It really annoyed me to hear them.

When I had our third baby, Asante, it was after I had had this experience in OB-GYN. As a matter of fact, his birth interrupted my clerkship in that area. I was furious just thinking what a terrible time those girls were having. The doctors would wait until the last minute to take them into the delivery rooms because they didn't want to just wait around with their hands gloved. In my opinion, the deliveries were chaos.

FORTUNATO: It's hard for me to discuss the benefits to us or to the baby specifically. It just seems like such a natural thing. People have had babies at home for a long time. We had confidence in Dr. Brew. There weren't any complications after little F.J. was born at home. We did feel there was some respiratory distress with Asante, but Dr. Brew and I took him to the hospital and had him checked by a neonatologist. Fortunately, the baby was OK so we brought him back home.

MARY: I definitely recommend home birth. I tell people who want to know about it that if you have a normal pregnancy and you've had a child before so that you know your pelvis is adequate, then there's no reason not to have the child at home. Being able to have your child in your own home, without hospital infections and nurses taking the child away, is really nice. Unfortunately, most people are skeptical. When I had my OB-GYN orals, the doctor said, "You've had a baby. Where did you have it?" I said, "I don't think I'll tell you because I'll get a bad grade." But he wanted to know and when I said, "At home," he said, "Wonderful!" That made me feel great.

Jeff and Elizabeth Record

ELIZABETH: I looked forward to having my babies at home. Having seen home deliveries as a part of my Peace Corps training, I had a very positive attitude about the whole procedure. We spent a week in the Chicago Maternity Center before we went to Malaysia. Asians do home deliveries all the time, and as I witnessed them, I began to appreciate the rightness of their ways. It was a stroke of luck to start to work for Dr. Brew—positive reinforcement. During the year that I was with him, I got to know patients who had had home deliveries and were just ecstatic about them.

JEFF: I was curious about the whole process. I had never seen a live birth before Jamie's, but I was assured by Dr. Brew that it was safe and a reasonable thing to do. As Elizabeth and I went through the childbirth training, I really became interested. I got the growing feeling that there was no reason to say goodbye to my wife at the door and then wait to hear that I'd become a father. It seemed to me that births should be a shared experience, and home birth was the answer for us.

ELIZABETH: For Jamie's birth, I knew I was in labor, but Jeff had an old college friend coming over for dinner. I had prepared a big pot of spaghetti and meatballs; and I was determined to sit down and eat dinner with them, even if I delivered right there in the middle of the diningroom! After I straightened up the kitchen, I went up and took another warm bath. In those last two weeks I had taken so many warm baths that I was beginning to feel like a prune. Then I got into bed and timed the contractions. The first labor, with Ian, had been manageable because it had been spaced out nicely over a long period of time. But the second one was easier because it was faster.

I think Jeffery was blasé about this one, since the last one had gone so well. Ian had seen me doing exercises every evening and would tell me when to pant, and so forth. I had shown Ian pictures of his own birth and told him about the coming of the new baby. Ian came into the room when I was in hard labor, but most of the time he spent with a family friend. He didn't happen to be there for the actual birth, but he did come in while Dr. Brew was suturing a little tear. I was smiling but breathing heavily. Ian was very curious about what Dr. Brew was doing.

I didn't want Ian to be whisked away from home during that period for the same reason I wouldn't go to the hospital and leave him. It would look to him as if he were kicked out because we had a new baby at our house. I had no qualms about his staying at home. Initally, he was very curious about the baby. He wanted to hold him and study him. After a few days Ian got a little combative, but at least he was verbalizing his feelings.

I liked having the baby with me from the moment of birth—not in a nursery. I've worked in a nursery. The routine was that if the babies cried in between

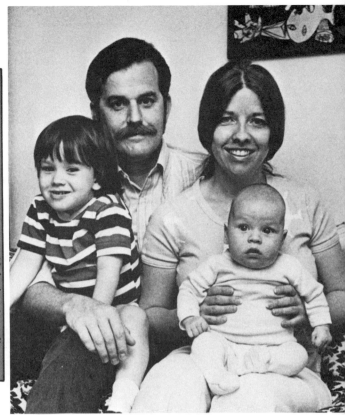

Elizabeth, 31, a graduate of Mount Auburn School of Nursing in Cambridge, Mass., joined the Peace Corps and served two years in Malaysia. Later she worked for Dr. Brew at his Yater Clinic office. Her husband, Jeff, 30, is a research associate at the Brookings Institution in Washington, D.C., where he specializes in analyzing European defense. Having recently written the *U.S. Force Structure in N.A.T.O: An Alternative*, Jeff is currently writing another book concerning tactical nuclear strategy. The Records reside in Silver Spring, Md., with their two young sons, 3-year-old Ian and 3-month-old James. Both boys were born at home with the assistance of Dr. Brew, and Janet Epstein.

the four-hour feeding schedule, we were supposed to give them a little boiled water and stick a pacifier into their mouths. They were all in those little beds lined up in a row. It's much nicer to have my baby close by where I can nurse it if I want to and see it all the time. If I'm at all apprehensive about the baby's condition, I have it right there where I can observe it closely, and I've got my husband there and our older boy—the family unit.

I feel our home births were very intimate experiences. Hospitals are for the convenience of the staff—the patients come second. Yet, when we tell our friends that we had two babies at home,

they're shocked. The general feeling is, "What if something goes wrong?" There are only negative reactions. Everyone we knew when we were first married went to the hospital, had plenty of drugs and didn't know what had happened to them. Jeff and I didn't want any part of that.

JEFF: I feel the increased disenchantment with doctors in general and the medical profession may be one of the reasons for natural childbirth and home deliveries. Some people just don't want to get involved with all the formality. Besides, I didn't want anyone hauling off my baby to a bland nursery to suck on a cold nipple and sugar water all alone!

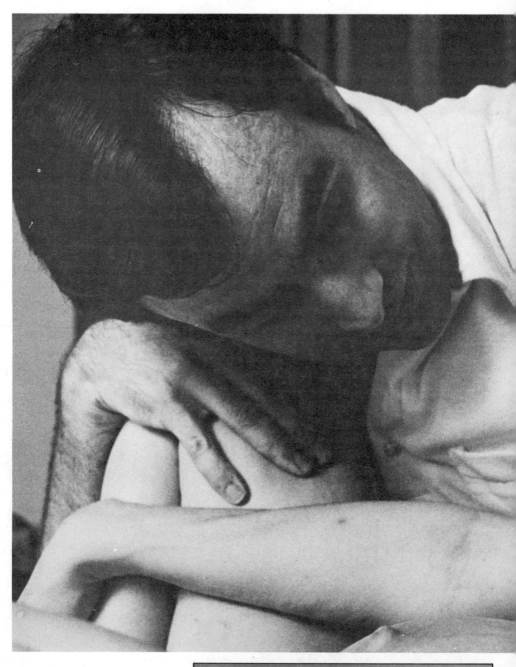

PHIL AND
LEE SIMON

Phil, 34, an engineer, and Lee, 32, a home-
maker and La Leche League Leader, shared the
medicated hospital birth of their first daughter,
Jennifer, 4. Photographed in their Crofton, Md.,
home, Carey's birth in May, 1975, was attended
by Nurse-midwife Janet Epstein.

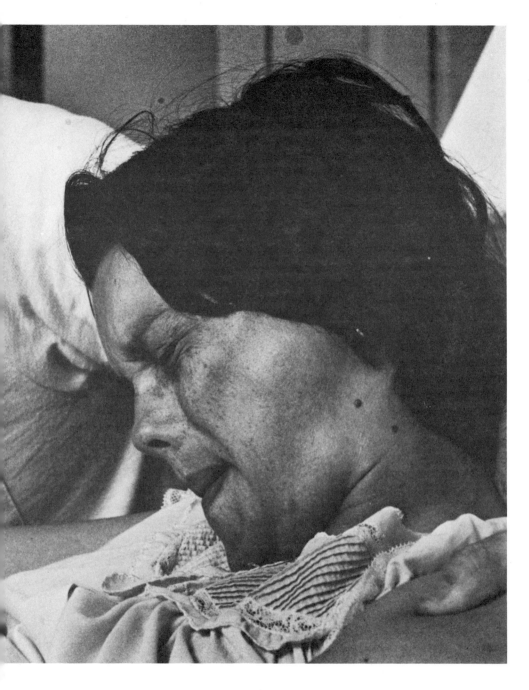

PHIL: Lee worked hard to get her home birth. She searched for months to find a doctor or a midwife. Never once did I feel she was in danger or worry about her. We never had any serious doubts that she could do it. The actual birth experience was worth all the effort. It's the most wonderful thing we have ever done.

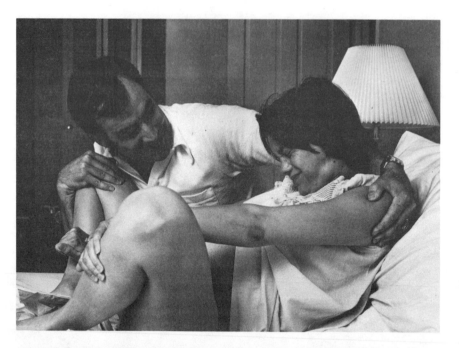

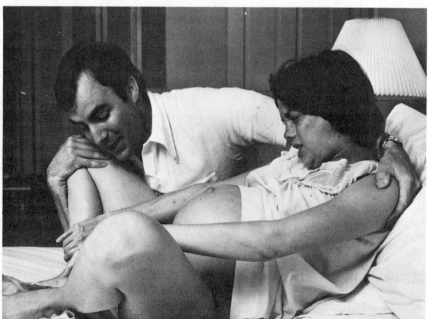

LEE: I was really touched by the simplicity of the birth, uncomplicated, in our own bed. Jan had out only some suture material and a sterile pair of scissors. We had a good working relationship. I felt we were integrated in our efforts. When I hesitated, Jan's voice came through clear and direct. She knew what I wanted, and I knew she wanted it for me. It was a tremendous feeling to trust someone like that when I needed support and concentration.

115

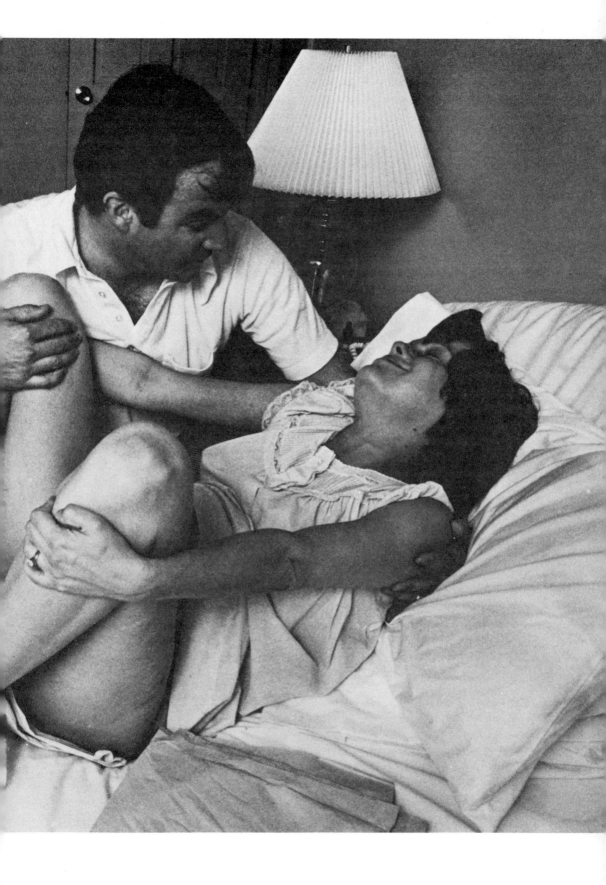

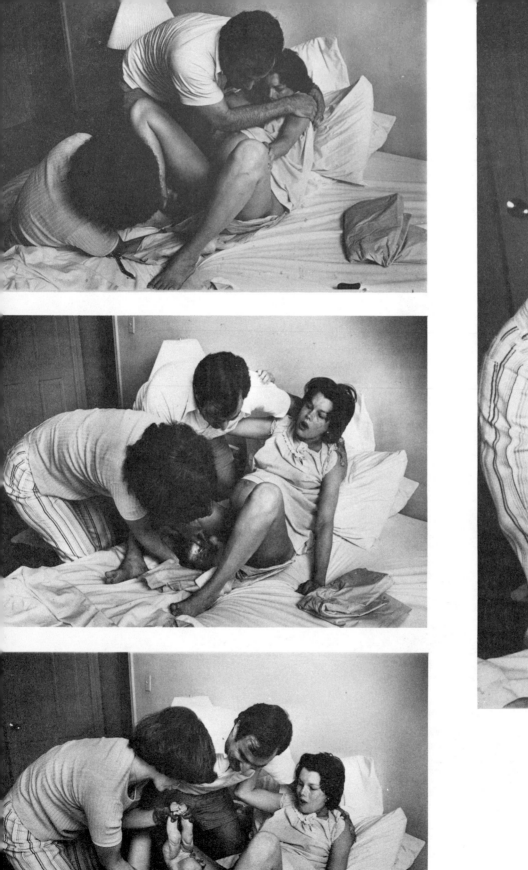
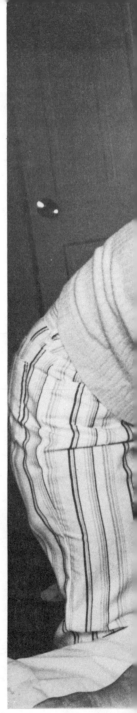

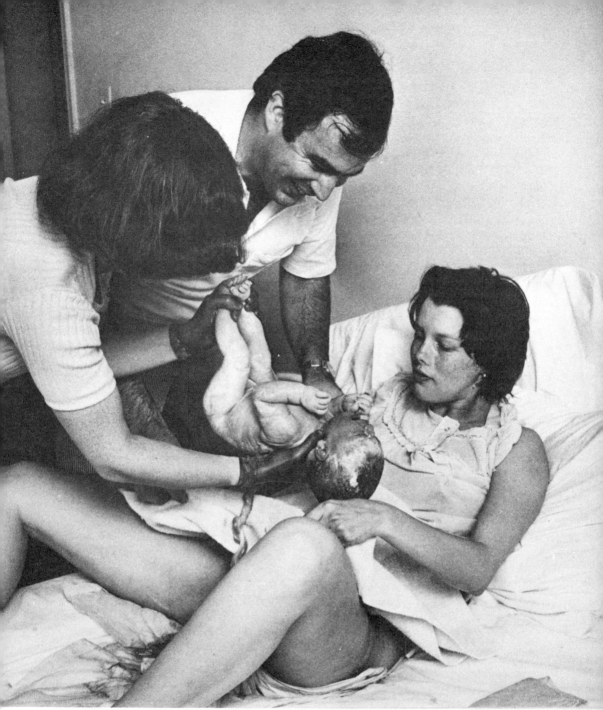

LEE: There was a lot going on between us. Phil literally picked me up with each contraction. He kept encouraging me. Suddenly I could see all the effort would soon be over. I don't know how I could ever have done it without him.

PHIL: Once the baby's head began to show, I became very excited. I remember seeing every hair on her head, then her face coming out, then her little hand right there. I was fascinated with the actual birth. The instant the baby was born, Lee's whole attitude changed. I could see it in her face. I felt extremely proud of her and the experience we had together.

118

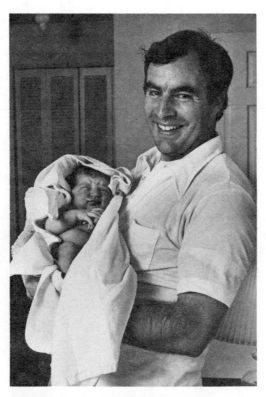

PHIL: This was the high point of my life.

LEE: Seeing the baby's vulnerability, I felt a rush of protectiveness. Having Carey in my arms was like a reward for all the times I had wanted to hold her. It was like, "Oh, here she is at last!"

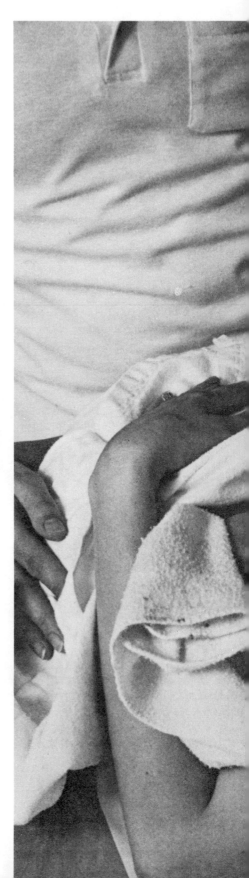

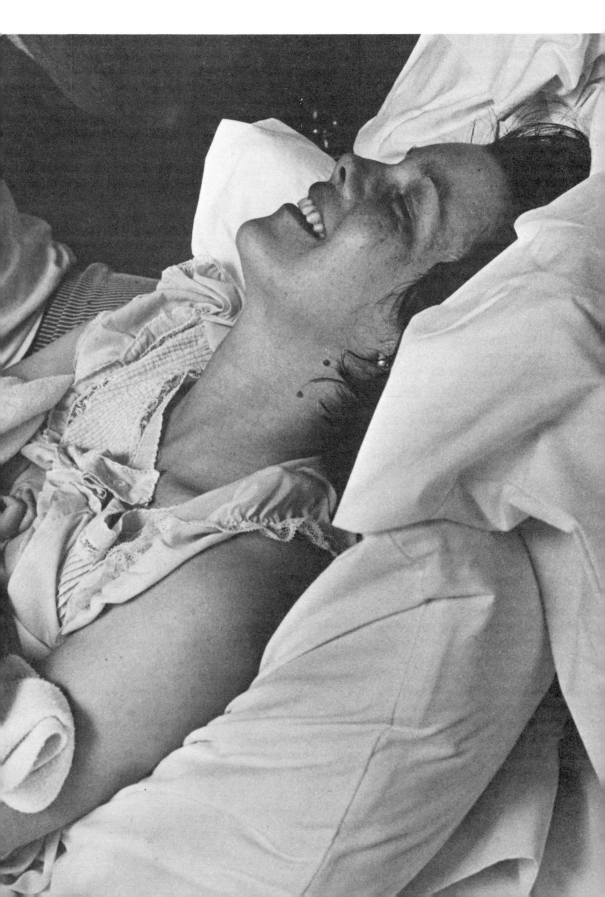

Mike and Jann Lamb

Jann, 20, calls herself a "full time working mother." After graduation from the same high school, Mike and Jann married in 1971. Now Mike, 19, works as a plumber. Having begun painting in school, Jann still pursues her hobby, preferring oils to acrylics. Two-and-a-half years ago Jason was born in the hospital with natural childbirth. The Lambs had Rachael Marie (right) in the apartment they are constructing beneath the home of Mike's parents in Rockville, Md. Dr. Brew and Nancy Knapp assisted in the birth. Jann's mother, Mary McIntyre, came down from her home in Mt. Airy, Md. While studying for a B.A. in sociology at Frederick Community College in Frederick, Md., Mary works as a psychiatric aide at Springfield State Hospital in Sykesville.

JANN: I have a friend who had her baby at home just before I had Jason. Her father and brother and husband delivered the baby. Everything seemed to work out nicely for her.

MARY (Jann's mother): They are friends of the family. When I went to see the baby, I told them, "It looks pretty good for a homemade baby!"

JANN: I had wanted to have Jason at home, but we didn't really have a home at the time. We were living upstairs with Mike's parents. So, I had Jason in the hospital. He had to be born somewhere.

I went through a clinic, and we didn't know a doctor who would deliver at home. The staff there were a lot of help in finding a childbirth class for us. With Jason, I had a very, very easy, quick birth.

MIKE: Jann woke me up first about 6:15.

JANN: I woke you up first about 3 A.M.

MIKE: I timed the contractions. They were very irregular and hard, so we went to the hospital right away. I was supposed to be present in the delivery room. The

121

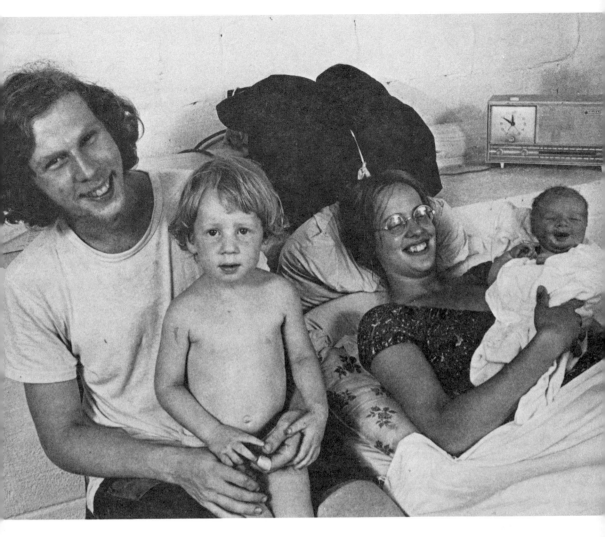

nurse told me to wait in the waiting room until Jann was prepared. I sat there about 45 minutes until they called me. I was expecting to go to the labor room. They said, "Right through these doors." There were Jann and Jason on the cot. I'd missed everything.

JANN: Jason was born at 7:45, about an hour and a half after we got up. I asked for Mike in the labor room. The nurse kept saying, "Oh, you don't really want to see him now, do you?" That's the only thing I asked for. They kept insisting, "Are you *sure* you don't want anything for the pain?" I said, "No, I don't want *any*thing." It seemed as if there were eighty-eight different nurses in and out and half of them couldn't have cared less about me. I just sort of figure I did it on my own.

MIKE: They wouldn't let Jann breast-feed the baby for the first twelve hours.

JANN: They said I couldn't have him because he had a little bit of mucus.

MIKE: But in the meantime, they were feeding him glucose water and formula out of a bottle. If he could drink *that*, why couldn't he nurse?

122

JANN: This one nurse explained to me, "Now you don't want us to get him out here and have him start choking. Then we'd just have to take him back. You don't want *that*, do you?" I didn't say anything because I didn't know what to say. I just wanted to see him. It wasn't the way I had wanted it to be.

I did eventually get to nurse Jason. He stopped when he was about fifteen months old.

MIKE: He was on a demand schedule, but he was pretty regular in his demands.

JANN: When I found out I was pregnant, I immediately started looking for a doctor who would deliver at home. I figured it would take me a while.

MIKE: I liked the idea of a home birth. At first Jann was talking about wanting to have a friend do it because she didn't know a doctor. I don't go along with it unless there is a doctor present. No matter how good Jann's health was, there was always a chance of a complication.

JANN: The clinic recommended Dr. Katherine Chapman. I went to her until three weeks ago when she had to drop out for her own health reasons. I started calling again until I found Nancy Knapp and Dr. Brew.

MARY: I was all for the home delivery. In fact, I'd always thought I'd like to have had my own babies at home, but I'm Rh-negative and the doctors wouldn't let me. I hated being in the hospital. The nurses were always after me to stay in bed, keep my shoes on if I walked around, and go to bed early. With six children, I've had a lot of hospital experience.

My mother had us at home. When I was six, my brother was born. I remem-ber that someone trundled me out of bed in the middle of the night to see him. I was so sleepy that I didn't have much of an impression of him that night. The next morning I thought he was really pretty cute.

When I was pregnant with Janet, my first, we didn't have any classes and no-body told us anything about what to expect. People didn't talk about natural childbirth then. Janet was the only one I had naturally. Even though everything turned out fine, the experience was a di-saster for me. After that I had medication with the others.

I guess that's why I didn't want to see the actual birth, but I am glad I was there in the house. Janet's very relaxed. She always just flows along.

JANN: I like it a lot better being at home. This birth took much longer than I expected, because Jason had been so fast. With him it wasn't nearly as hard as this labor with Rachael. I got so tired by the end. I don't know if I would have *made* it this time without Mike.

MIKE: I was pretty tired emotionally and physically, but I thought it was really exciting. Not many people witness the birth of their own child, which is some-thing I'll always remember. I enjoyed participating, and I feel I had a very defi-nite part.

JANN: He has bruises on his arms and knees where I hung on.

MIKE: And a couple of deep gouges.

I saw Jason only for a few seconds when he was half an hour old. Then I didn't see him again except through a plate glass window until three days later. He was really different from the first time I saw him. This way, the change is more gradual. I can note the progress as it takes place. I hold the baby quite a bit, and in the middle of the night, after Jan wakes me up, I bring the baby to her so she won't have to get out of bed.

JANN: With Jason, I got to see him when he was just born, all grey and "yucky;" then they wrapped him up and I got to hold him for a few minutes. The next time I saw him he had completely changed. With Rachael, all of a sudden here's the baby and I can take care of her. At first I could see how she was attached to me. I've gotten to see her navel the whole time, while with Jason, the cord had dried up by the time I got him home. Not that the navel is anything so *marvelous*, but it is a *detail*.

MARY: Rachael changed color like a color TV out of whack. She was purple in the face, lavender in the hands, red in the back. And within an hour after birth, she was a little pink and white baby.

JANN: I was glad not to have to wait until visiting hours to see Mike and the rest of my family. And I was glad we didn't have to find somebody to keep Jason while I was in the hospital. We didn't want Jason in the room for the birth though.

MIKE: If he had been old enough to know what was going on, then it would have been a good thing, but he's still so young, only two-and-a-half.

JANN: After everyone left our house that night, I got up and changed clothes. Then Mike and I stayed awake and talked for a long time.

MIKE: We were able to talk about the birth and compare notes, whereas, in the hospital, I could only see Jann for a few minutes at a visit. Then, by the time she came home, I'd forgotten what I wanted to say before or the time for saying it had passed. It was really nice to be together after Rachael's birth.

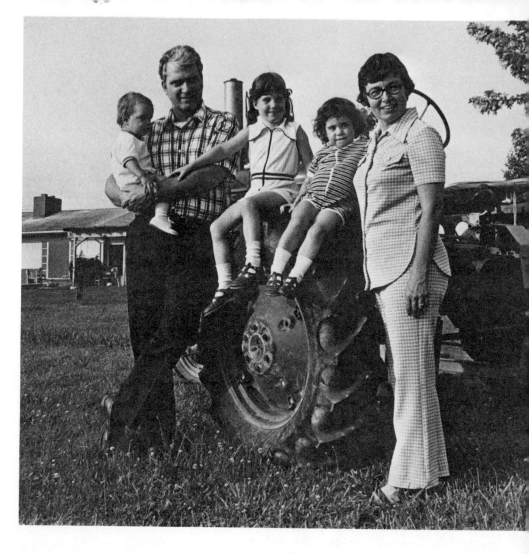

Carol and Chris Noonan

Carol, 45, and Chris, 40, and their three little girls live in Rockville, Md. Kit, 5, was born in the hospital with prepared childbirth. Meg, 2½, and Carol Ann, 15 months, were both born at home. Before starting her family, Carol worked in the Montgomery County school system as a special education teacher. Chris is a mechanical engineer working at the U.S. Navy Research and Development Center. Dr. Katharine Chapman, a general practitioner, since retired, and Janet Epstein, attended the home births.

CAROL: We wanted to have our first baby at home, but Dr. Chapman doesn't do that, especially since I was older, 40 at the time, and had no obstetrical history.

CHRIS: As it turned out, we easily could have. We just about had Kit in Dr. Chapman's office.

CAROL: She'd just gotten back from another delivery and her tools weren't ready.

CHRIS: After we got to the doctor's office, she told me, "Look, there's the baby's head." I said, "Hey, you're right." As we were driving to the hospital, I remember thinking, "This is ridiculous—and dangerous."

CAROL: Her last instructions to me were, "Don't push." I thought, "Ha, ha!" but we made it. After they separated Chris and me, they sent me right to the delivery room. They were all standing around wondering what to do. I was four hours in the delivery room. The doctor admitted that it was just psychological. Being separated from Chris was quite traumatic. I think I was concerned over what he was going through, when I should have had my full attention on giving birth.

CHRIS: Yeah, that was tough. Since it took so long, I had just about come to the conclusion that they were both dead in there. This is insane, yet people go through this on a regular basis—they wait too late—when they could be relaxed and have it at home with no problems—or a minimum of problems.

CAROL: I really don't have any horror stories about the hospital. It just was sort of a nuisance. I went in and delivered and came home the next day. Of course, Chris and I were separated. It's sort of dumb. When you get to that stage and they say, "You go that way, and we'll go this." I found it very disturbing when they took my baby away—even when I knew it was going to happen. Being separated from my baby right after it was born was a terrible emotional trauma.

CHRIS: Another reason we wanted to have our second child at home was because we didn't want to go off and leave our first child, Kit. Dr. Chapman said right away that the next child could be born at home. The only interesting thing about this birth was that Meg was a posterior presentation and weighed eight and a half pounds. I've had doctors

tell me since then that I couldn't have done it at home. It was hard pushing, and I did have an episiotomy.

CHRIS: It's a good thing that Dr. Chapman was there to catch Meg. She shot out so fast—she literally shot out. She came out crying, so she had a perfect score on her Apgar test. I was curious about what the placenta looked like, but I couldn't tell much about it. I took it out and buried it in our garden. I was curious about what my own reactions would be to the whole process, with slight apprehension, but I was so busy—the chief "go-fer," you know. I didn't have much time to think.

CAROL: Chris did everything as if he'd rehearsed the whole affair. He gave a marvelous performance. It just seemed as though everyone was moving as if he were in a play, and I felt like the star. Just at the right time, Chris came around and sat by my head, when I needed someone to hold on to. This was very comforting to me. I always wondered what you hold on to. What I held on to was Chris's hand, which was far superior to bars. About two pushes and the baby was born. I really didn't have time to think ethereal thoughts. It just happened as it was supposed to. Sometimes I worried afterward that it wasn't dramatic enough.

CHRIS: Just the quiet peace of it all. That's the drama.

CAROL: After Meg was born, I couldn't get back to sleep. My adrenalin was up so high. And then there's nothing to do once the baby's all tucked up and sleeping, so Chris went out to get the newspaper for me.

CHRIS: Animals seem to know intuitively what we are only now relearning. Our dog, Gretel, gave birth to puppies not long after Meg arrived. It was like she had gone to a Lamaze course. She started off her labor with a deep heavy slow breathing. As it increased, her breathing picked up its pace; and as she delivered, there was panting. She looked so fatigued and bothered at this point. Since I'd just been through the course, I figured, "This is all so similar. I'm going to get her some ice chips." And you should have seen the look on her face, like, "Oh, this is *exactly* what I wanted!" Like she was a Lamaze student. Here this "dumb" animal instinctively knows what we're trying to teach our allegedly sophisticated people—what they've lost through this medical brainwashing technique over the centuries. Since then, I've talked to people on farms and apparently this is how it's done in nature. It's really a shame we've lost it, but I guess we're getting it back slowly.

CAROL: As for Carol Ann's birth, there's almost no story. My labor was so short, an hour and a half.

CHRIS: Carol fooled me. She said, "Call the doctor." But at that time, judging from the other two births, I figured there was no hurry. I was timing contractions, but one or two particular contractions don't tell the whole story.

CAROL: He wanted to be able to give a good report when he called the doctor. I guess she knew because she said, "I'll be right over."

CHRIS: Actually Jan made it, well, *half* made it. I noticed some headlights coming into the driveway. Carol said, "Uh, oh!" and I saw the baby's head.

CAROL: Chris's classic comment was, "Wait a minute."

CHRIS: It was either go to the door for Jan or quickly review my birth-delivery instructions. As it was, Jan just came in and looked and said, "Push," so she finished the delivery and I said, "Gee, why didn't I think of that? I could have had it all to myself and she took all the glory!" Dr. Chapman arrived a few minutes later.

I have never been enthusiastic about giving birth in a hospital. We took the tour before Kit was born, and when I walked into their stainless steel cell, I couldn't believe that people go into those things. But I guess most don't know what a choice they have.

The psychological and physical aspects of birth are so intertwined, the psychological being extremely dominant, in my opinion. Good old medicine has so distorted the process. I guess it reached its peak in the infamous twilight sleep days. It just wiped a woman out. What the psychological aspect of the relaxed home atmosphere comes down to, is that if she wants two thousand pillows, she gets two thousand pillows, and if she wants ice, she gets ice. Also, with the hospital delivery, when Mommy goes away, she comes back with a baby. That adds to the mystique about sex and babies. The child comes from the mother. How much more basic can you get than that? The advantages are total to the family. We've never slept apart from the children. It's so subtle an effect—having the family solidified rather than separated. The other children were so young when Carol Ann was born. It's hard to say what they got out of it all, but maybe that in itself is good. Because the other way, they might remember the separation and the bad parts; this way, if there is any memory, it's just a part of family life.

127

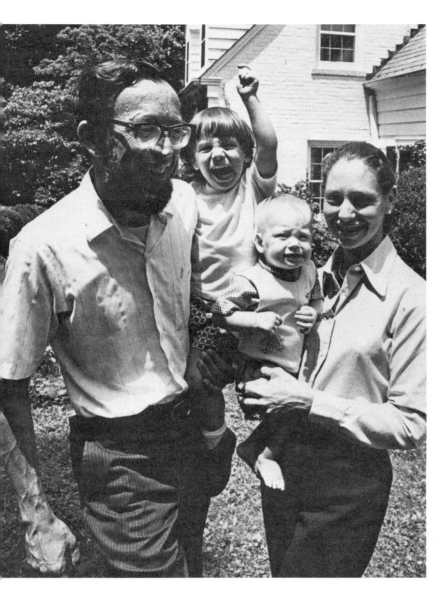

Miriam
and
Ed Kelty

Miriam and Ed, who both hold doctorates in psychology, chose to have both of their children by home birth.* Joel is 2½ years old and Ruth was born ten months ago in the Kelty home in Bethesda, Md. In attendance were Dr. Brew and Janet Epstein.

*(See ''The Psychological Dimension,'' pp. 61-64.)

MIRIAM: I spoke with a friend, also a psychologist, who works with infants and is a professor of obstetrics and gynecology at Georgetown University. I asked her to refer me to three very different obstetricians. One was a very conservative gentleman. He immediately did assorted lab work on me, told me that I shouldn't carry the groceries but that it was all right to walk, gave me a very quaint book with a personal inscription and a variety of instructions. He said that he would deliver the baby by whatever method I wanted, but that he didn't think much of natural childbirth. Dr. Brew was the second physician I saw. The third was thoroughly nondescript. Of the three, Dr. Brew was the only one who didn't treat pregnancy as a disease; this fit my own philosophy perfectly.

I did not go shopping for home delivery. I did actively seek a physician whom I felt was competent and compatible and one who would respect my wishes. I wanted a natural unmedicated birth. In the course of conversation during my second or third visit, Dr. Brew mentioned that he did home deliveries. I said, "You must have a lot of confidence in yourself," and he cited his experience and statistics. I said, "Ok, I'll take one of those." Among the reasons for wanting the baby to be born at home were my husband's and my attitude toward pregnancy and birth. We feel they are normal processes and highly personal life experiences. Also, we've both worked in enough hospitals that we don't have automatic respect for them and trust in them.

My pregnancy was uneventful. I was in good physical condition. I started to swim when I was pregnant—about a half mile a day. Ed and I felt well informed about pregnancy, birth, and newborns. I did ask Dr. Brew to show me how to determine the position of the baby, where the head and where the rear were, so I felt confident that the baby was not breech. Ed and I did our homework. We read extensively and felt prepared to deliver the baby ourselves if we had to.

Joel was born on a Sunday night. We had a very uneventful pleasant labor. It was practically over by the time I thought it was going to hurt. I had about three very painful contractions and thought that they were the beginning of about forty-five minutes' worth; however, that was it.

ED: You said, "Now I guess the real thing is going to begin," and Dr. Brew said, "No, that's over." You were thirsty and wanted a drink. You said, "When am I going to feel nauseous?" Dr. Brew said, "Well, that time has passed, too."

MIRIAM: We were tremendously impressed that Dr. Brew arrived at our home dressed for a weekend evening, and that he kept his jacket on and his sleeves buttoned until the baby was practically born. This effectively communicated to me that the delivery wasn't going to be a bloody mess.

ED: His white shirt was as clean when he finished as when he started. He himself commented that he wonders why it's so sloppy in the hospital.

MIRIAM: I said that I didn't want an episiotomy if I didn't need one. Janet and Dr. Brew said it depended on me, on how much control I had. At one point, Dr. Brew asked me if I could wait a minute and not push. He slowed the emergence of the baby's head for two contractions, and that was that. I did not have an episiotomy. It all went extremely well. We were very happy. After Joel was born, everybody stayed here for about two hours and drank champagne out of long-stemmed glasses.

The nicest part was that after Dr. Brew and Janet left, Ed and I walked back to our own bed and cuddled up—the three of us! Had I been in a hospital, feeling so elated, so wide awake and all, I would have been very intolerant, I'm sure. By the next morning I would have probably marched myself outside for a walk or some such thing.

ED: So the next morning Miriam came down and made breakfast. Then her mother flew in and was very surprised when Miriam met her at the door. The Tuesday after the baby was born on Sunday was the last Childbirth Education Association class in the series we attended. The nurses called up and said, "Would you please come to the class and bring the baby?" I said, "It's snowing out there!" but they told me it wouldn't make any difference as far as the baby was concerned and it would be so wonderful for the class. So we packed ourselves up and went to tell our classmates how it went. What impressed them was that Miriam was walking around wearing her regular clothes and not being an invalid.

I think that the variables involved in the birth experience going so well were: first, Miriam felt comfortable and positive about this kind of a relationship and our decision; it was useful to be informed by going to C.E.A. classes and reading; second, she was in top-notch physical condition because she swam and did the childbirth preparation exercises faithfully.

MIRIAM: I went to see Dr. Brew *before* I became pregnant the second time to make sure that he wasn't going to be away on vacation when the next baby would probably be born. Ruth's birth was also planned to occur at a convenient time in relation to our jobs. We decided to have our children very close together in age.

Toward the end of another very uneventful pregnancy, Ed and I had the opportunity to participate in a week-long meeting in Santa Cruz, Calif. Two-and-a-half weeks before the baby was due, I went to see Dr. Brew and said, "I know that it may be crazy, but it's been a very, very hectic summer, and it's enticing to go to Santa Cruz." I realized that the baby might be born in California, but I didn't anticipate any problems. Dr. Brew's attitude was that it was really a matter of how much dependency I wanted to have toward him. He gave me the name of a friend who was competent but who was not an advocate of natural childbirth. Dr. Brew told me that almost everywhere in California husbands are allowed in the delivery rooms and that it would be up to us from that point on to fight for what we wanted. Knowing us, he said, we would probably fight hard and get our way.

After we got to Santa Cruz, we arranged for contingency facilities and went through the week's conference without event. I started to bleed a little Friday night. After being checked by a local physician and calling Dr. Brew, we decided that we would return home on Saturday night. Both Janet and Dr. Brew felt that there would be no great difficulty in delivering on the airplane, if it came to that. We took the overnight plane so that Joel could sleep. It was an uneventful flight home, except that Joel preferred exploring the plane to sleeping.

On Sunday afternoon, a friend called and invited us to his new house for a drink. It was hot, so we decided that sounded terrific and went. At this point I was feeling uncomfortable enough so that I couldn't sit down for very long, but I was not experiencing any timeable contractions. We came back home about 5:30. I made Joel dinner, gave him a bath, and put him to bed. Then I started changing the bed and rounding up a bowl for the placenta, blankets, and newspapers. After everything was in order, we called Janet. She was planning to go out to dinner and wanted to finish baking a blueberry pie she was to take with her. We said, "Yes," but twenty minutes later, I called back and said, "I'm not particularly uncomfortable, in which case this may all be a mistake, *or* the baby is going to be born very soon." Janet came right over, and Dr. Brew arrived soon after. I was about nine centimeters dilated and quite comfortable. I wasn't even using any of the breathing techniques. Dr. Brew ruptured the membranes and said, "Don't you have an irresistible urge to push?" And I said, "No." "You'd better push if you want to see that baby." About three pushes later, there was Ruth! She just popped out.

We collectively did her Apgar rating. She got a 9½ out of the possible 10. Her feet could have been pinker, but she was clearly very healthy. I wasn't at all tired, except from jet lag. It was such a fast delivery that it wasn't exhausting at all.

ED: Ruth was born at 8:10 P.M. so that both Dr. Brew and Janet were able to make their evening social engagements. They left about twenty minutes after the birth, so we knew that they had absolutely no anxiety about our wellbeing.

Our parents had been somewhat more concerned than we were before Joel was born. In fact, they were very much opposed to the whole notion of home delivery. But once they accepted the fact that this is what we were going to do, we learned that most of them had been born at home, too. And Uncle Harry, a physician, had delivered a number of babies at home. He had just wisely withheld comment until it was quite clear our minds were made up.

I certainly appreciated the home approach. There are differences in people, which we recognize. Some think the new mother's entitled to a good week's rest after the hard work of delivery. Our own feeling is that we'd rather take the week's rest at a pleasant place, not the hospital. After all, there are resorts that are designed to cater to people's needs to be pampered much more effectively than a hospital can.

MIRIAM: After each birth, we both stayed home from work for a week just enjoying ourselves and getting to know our new baby.

ED: Miriam and I liked the closeness, the non-artificiality of the experience. We didn't have to be involved with other people at a time when we wanted to interact with each other. It was a lot easier just to work from our own feelings of how we wanted it done.

We have received first class treatment from competent professionals at home without any of the bright, shiny hospital equipment, which deludes people into thinking they're being modern. We feel childbirth is a normal developmental process and that home is the healthiest place for it—physically and emotionally.

Home Birth assures closesness between siblings from the very beginning of life for the newborn. And the older child feels no loss of love when allowed to be a participant in this most important of family events.

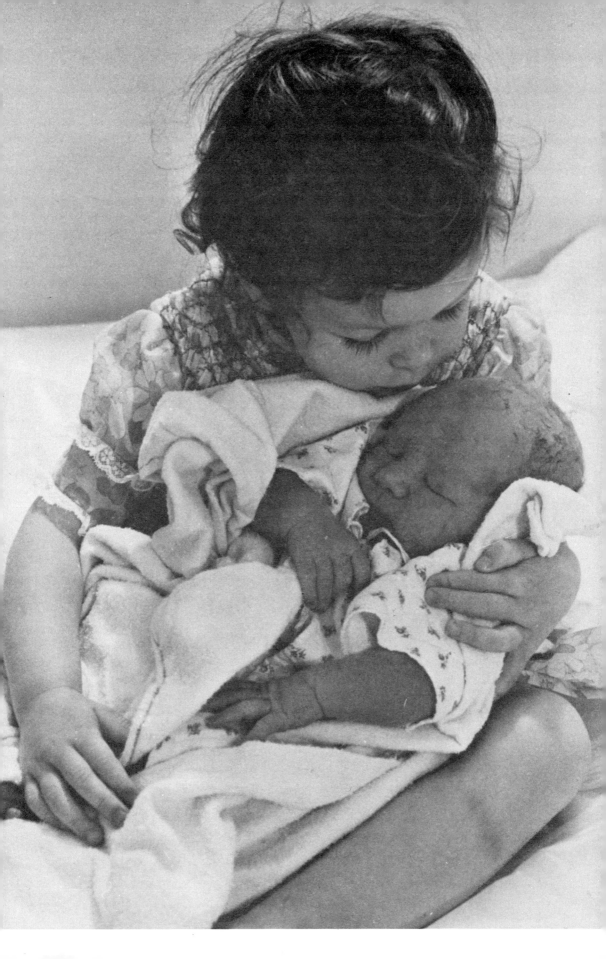

Home Birth in America

an overview
by Charlotte Ward

At one time, all human births were home births. Until a few decades ago the overwhelming majority of American babies were born in their mothers' beds. Today such births in this country are enjoyed by only a select few. This overview will trace that pendulum swing from birth at home to hospital confinements; it then notes that a new swing is now underway which will hopefully bring a new era of home births.

Home Birth in the 1700s and 1800s

Early American babies arrived in forts, in flatboats on the broad rivers, in covered wagons, and in trains. A few came in big-city "lying-in" establishments, already widespread in Europe, but the vast majority of eighteenth and nineteenth century babies were born at home. Attendants included the husband, the other womenfolk of the family, and often, the fathers-in-law, too. Doctors were sent for when they were available, but the Southern colonial pioneer also put much stock in the "granny woman," a midwife usually equipped with little more than a clean apron, years of experience, and a few herbs.

Women faced birth realistically; they had witnessed and had themselves felt the pleasures and the pain connected with birth in their families. In her book, *Flowering of the Cumberland*, Harriette Arnow observes that in her research she found no evidence of maternity-associated mental illness or of child abuse. Most new mothers, with rare exception, could suckle their children, the major reason for a high percentage of success being that the mother and child were seldom separated from each other. These farmers' wives were well aware that a newborn calf or lamb could not be taken from its mother for long without serious results—either abandonment by the mother or death of the young.

There was generally a great deal of support and seasoned advice available to the first-time mother, and all childbearing women must have been considerably helped by the two-week "lying-in period" deemed necessary for their rest and recuperation. Tucked in beside her, the new baby was treated in a warm and deferential manner and nursed at his whim. Indeed, the baby continued to get this kind of attention, or until his mother got pregnant again, for two or three years.

The greater the distance from civilization, the harder life became for the frontiersmen and their families. Fewer doctors, insufficient knowledge and equipment, longer distances, as well as limited diets and harsh conditions made childbirth an often feared and very dangerous occurrence. Histories make scant mention of maternity per se, usually noting only the most unusual stories. However, a few accounts do exist that give us a glimpse of normal childbirth in the pioneer setting. One such diary is that of Mary Walker, a missionary lady in the Oregon territory who is reputed to have been the third white woman to cross the Rockies. On December 7, 1838, she wrote:

Awoke about five o'clock. As soon as I moved was surprised by discharge which I supposed indicated approaching confinement. Felt unwilling it should happen in the absence of my husband. I waited a few moments. Soon pains began to come on, and I sent Mrs. Smith who lodged with me to call Mrs. Whitman. She came and called her husband. They made what preparations they deemed necessary, and left to attend worship and breakfast, after which or about nine I became quite sick enough. Began to feel discouraged. Felt as if I almost wished I had never been married. But there was no retreating, meet it I must. About eleven I began to be quite discouraged. I had hoped to be delivered ere then. I was so tired, and knew nothing, how long before I should be relieved. But just as I supposed the worst was at hand, my ears were saluted with the cry of my child. "A son" was the salutation. Soon I forgot my misery in the joy of possessing a proper child. Surely I felt to say with Eve "I have gotten a man from the Lord," or with Hannah "For this child I prayed." Thanks to a kind Providence for so great and unmerited a blessing. The remainder of the day I was comfortable. Husband returned in the evening with a thankful heart, I trust, and plenty of kisses for me and my boy. Mrs. Smith stayed with me through the night, her husband being gone from home.

Although the birth itself was without complications, Mary did suffer terribly from a breast infection. This could have meant starvation for her baby had not another missionary mother and an Indian mother helped to supplement her own diminished milk supply. Mary went on to bear seven more children. Of a later birth she writes:

Rested well last night; awoke about four a.m. Rose at five, helped about milking, but by the time I had done that, found it necessary to call my husband and soon the Dr. Had scarcely time to dress and comb my hair. Before eight was delivered of a fine daughter.

Once Mary tells of answering the doctor's knock at the door with her new baby already in her arms. Another entry reads:

Rose about five. Had early breakfast. Got my house work done about nine. Baked six loaves of bread. Made a kettle of mush and have now a suet pudding and beef boiling. My girl [an Indian helper] has ironed and I have managed to put my clothes away and set my house in order. May the merciful be with me through the unexpected scene. Nine o'clock p.m. was delivered of another son.

Later, as the prairie schooners plied their way westward, a broad range of rituals and events of family took place under the billowing canvasses. Sometimes the wagon trains were able to stop only long enough for the actual birth to be accomplished before moving steadily onward again. Surely these childbearing women were most in jeopardy—given the strains of their alien surroundings in addition to the jolting and unrelenting ride.

Gradually the vast Midwest was homesteaded and settled. Even then, birth continued to be hazardous. Food was often scarce, balanced and consistent nutrition being a virtual impossibility. The climatic conditions were severe both summer and winter, and the cramped sod houses and leantos were drafty and leaky.

A woman might well go into labor during a flood in the summer or a blizzard in the winter. Travel was difficult and uncertain. The few doctors who were available were hard put to answer all their requests or, once committed, meet their obligations. On the surface, the doctor's fee of that day appears small—fifty cents a mile for travel and one dollar for his call. But owing to the long distances he had to cover and the high price of the medicine he brought with him, his bill could easily reach $25. One woman, without the necessary $35 in cash, gave her doctor a heifer calf in partial payment, and then, having nothing else but her feather bed, offerd that for the remainder.

Because of the high cost and the fact that the baby often arrived before the doctor, many families did not go for a doctor at all. Neighbor women served as best they could in the midwife's role, and managed to look after the older children and help with the housework as much as their own work-burdened lives permitted. That left a substantial burden on the husband, already responsible for heavy ranch duties. During the period of confinement, and for months after if his wife were debilitated by the delivery, the husband also had to assume the household chores, cooking, childcare, and nursing his recuperating wife. These isolated families would certainly have been less vulnerable to maternity-associated illnesses and death had they been able to obtain a modicum of pre- and post-natal care.

Home Birth in the 1900s

By the early 1900s the lot of most child-bearing women remained unchanged. This is illustrated in a U.S. Department of Labor survey conducted between 1914 and 1918 to determine the quality of maternity care available to rural women. The investigators assured a cross-section of typical mothers by selecting seven counties in five states. During this period most Americans still lived in rural areas, rendering this study applicable to a large segment of the American people.

Although the occupations and the backgrounds of the various county populations surveyed were diverse, the maternity and childcare customs and problems were basically the same. Both husbands

and wives worked long, hard days on the farms. Many women in all areas had responsibilities for the poultry, gardening, and milking in addition to cooking, washing, and caring for their children. In most cases, the only mechanical convenience in the house was a sewing machine. Water usually had to be carried from an outside source, and outdoor privies and open disposal of waste water and garbage probably greatly degraded health.

The worst county record was in Montana, where homesteaders occupied 5,500 square miles without a hospital. Only three registered physicians worked in the whole state. The maternal mortality rate (deaths associated with pregnancy and birth) was 12.7 per 1,000; the infant mortality rate (babies who succumbed during their first year of life) was estimated at 91 per 1,000. About one-fifth of the women surveyed had been able to afford to leave home for a hospital delivery or at least a confinement among family or friends in a more populated community. But the cost of leaving was very high, from $150 to $700, so most women found home birth to be their only option.

The Kansas county reflected the most favorable statistics: Maternal mortality —2.9 per 1,000; infant mortality—40 per 1,000 live births. It is perhaps significant that 95 percent of these births were attended by physicians, since Kansas had no provisions for licensing midwives. Although there were three hospitals in the county, only ten country mothers had gone to them for childbirth during the two-year survey period. Hospital maternity care was generally regarded as a last resort. In Kansas and all other counties studied, prenatal and postnatal checkups were deemed "inadequate" in all but a handful of cases, and most mothers received no maternity-associated medical attention whatsoever.

135

Midwifery was the mainstay of the Southern counties of Mississippi, Tennessee, and North Carolina and in the Polish community of northern Wisconsin. Most of the "granny women" had no formal training in nursing, and some in the South could not even read and write. Although many of them made a conscious effort toward cleanliness in the birth procedures, few were equipped to handle emergencies. Still, many of the women interviewed expressed a definite preference for the midwives.

Most rural women expected many pregnancies during their childbearing years. Almost all of them had their first babies before they were 20 and got pregnant again every two or three years thereafter. Breastfeeding, initiated in over 99 percent of the births surveyed, made a positive contribution to childspacing and to children's nutrition. Table food was normally introduced around the fourth to the sixth month, and continued at least until the end of the first year. On the average, approximately one-fourth of the babies in all counties studied were still nursing at 18 months, and a considerable number past their second birthdays.

While the 1915 level of maternity care in the rural areas of our country was terribly inadequate by today's standards, the mortality statistics were lower than comparable figures for urban areas in those same states at that time. Childbirth in America had shown little substantial progress in safety since the country was first colonized.

Chicago Maternity Center

When Dr. Joseph B. DeLee returned to Chicago in 1895 from his studies in Vienna, he found an alarming maternal mortality rate of 4 out of every 1,000 births and an even higher infant mortality rate. By founding the Maxwell Street Dispensary, later known as the Chicago Maternity Center, he began to deliver children in a section of the city that had previously been midwife territory. By 1932, the Dispensary was delivering 3,600 babies a year at home, mostly to indigent patients. The majority preferred having their babies at home because they felt more in control of the situation and could continue to care for their other children. Also, the Visiting Nurses Association attended them for several weeks after birth.

Through the years, social welfare agencies, Northwestern University Medical School, and Chicago Medical School have participated in the Center's citywide service. The home births used to be employed as a training experience. Medical teams that went into each home consisted of a nurse-midwife, a student nurse, and two medical students, one of whom actually delivered the baby. In case of an emergency, a traveling resident specializing in obstetrics and gynecology immediately joined them, or the woman was transferred to the hospital. After 80 years of service, the Chicago Maternity Center (CMC) had delivered 150,000 babies, approximately 90 percent of them at home.

The CMC story vividly illustrates what has been happening on the home birth scene. Requests for home births dwindled from 300 to 30 a month by 1973, at which point it became unprofitable to continue the service. Now, all CMC deliveries and teaching take place in the hospital.

Maternity Center Association

Following in the footsteps of the Chicago Maternity Center, another big-city group concerned with better maternity care was established. In 1918 the Maternity Center Association (MCA) began to organize and operate a network of prenatal clinics throughout New York City. Their initial work showed an encouraging decrease in maternal and neonatal deaths among the women they taught and cared for. Then, when other agencies joined the educational and service arena, MCA chose a central Harlem district with a largely Spanish-speaking population on which to concentrate its efforts. Few of the women had been seeking or receiving adequate prenatal care. MCA aimed to develop "a complete maternity nursing service—ante-, intra-, and postpartal."

From the beginning MCA has been involved in education of the public and professionals alike. They believe that a better informed expectant mother and father will take more responsibility for themselves and have a safer birth experience. The staff has stressed the importance of a good diet, taught sewing classes, published books, held seminars, sponsored guest speakers, and championed prepared childbirth classes.

With the establishment in 1931 of the first nurse-midwifery school in the United States, a program of home deliveries could then be offered to the women of the Harlem district. Pregnant women were examined and any abnormalities referred to an obstetrician. At the onset of labor, a nurse-midwife and a student nurse went to the home and stayed with the woman until after her baby was born and everything was in order. In case of an emergency, the clinic physician was immediately consulted and appropriate action taken. Medical backup was provided by the Women's clinic of the New York Hospital.

The system worked well. There were no maternal deaths after 1939, when antibiotics came into use. In the period from 1932 to 1957, 7,000 women were delivered with a maternal mortality rate of .4 per 1,000. Eighty-eight percent of these 7,000 women had had home births; the remaining 12 percent had been hospitalized for medical reasons. The neonatal mortality rate was 15 per 1,000 live births.

In their publication, *Twenty Years of Nurse-Midwifery: 1933 - 1953*, MCA makes the following statement:

In the home delivery service associated with the school, it was shown that children could be born safely at home if the mothers and homes were carefully chosen, and that the resultant satisfactions contributed to greater relaxation and comfort during labor, greater security for mothers and children, and better family living.

In the years after that report, requests for home confinements decreased significantly. When the women in their district had originally refused to leave their homes for childbirth, MCA had responded with a home birth program. Again responding to their district, MCA discontinued its home birth program in 1958 and transferred its field service for nurse-midwifery education to Kings County Hospital in a joint program with the Hospital and State University of New York.

Marion Strachan, a consultant at MCA, stated that there has been a revival of interest in home births in the last five years. Requests now coming in are from a different socio-economic group. According to Ms. Strachan, middle income expectant parents are now seeking to have their babies at home.

Frontier Nursing Service

With the goal of lessening the rural isolation of Leslie County in eastern Kentucky, Mary Breckinridge founded the Frontier Nursing Service (FNS) in 1925. As a nurse-midwife, she devoted a major part of her 84 years to making life better for the children of the area. When she arrived not a single doctor practiced in the county and no roads penetrated the area. The nurse-midwives on the staff were obliged to ride horseback and carry their equipment in their saddlebags.

By 1939 FNS had grown sufficiently that it opened Frontier Graduate School of Nurse-Midwifery, thereby training more nurses to carry on family nursing care. Today FNS owns and operates the fully staffed 25-bed Hyden Hospital, the only one in the county, and mans six nursing stations at strategic points in the 1,000 square miles of rugged mountainous terrain. The nurses no longer travel by horseback; they use jeeps to reach the people.

Through the years the nurse-midwives and their trainees have given consistent and quality maternity care to the Kentucky hillfolk. They have many stories to tell that illustrate not only the life they lead but the spirit in which they pursue their work.

Frontier Nursing Service has now delivered almost 20,000 babies. Statistics are available for the first 10,000 births, which occurred between 1925 and 1955. Three-fourths of these births took place at home in settings that offered less than ideal conditions. The large proportion of teenage mothers and women who had had several babies make the following results even more impressive. By 1955 FNS had achieved a maternal mortality rate of .9 per 1,000 as compared to the U.S. rate for white women of the same period of 3.4 per 1,000 births. There has not been a maternal death at FNS since 1952. An average of the first 4,000 deliveries yielded a neonatal (first month of life) mortality rate of 30 per 1,000. The last 1,000 confinements of the first 10,000 compared very positively; the neonatal mortality rate for this group was down to 17.3 as against the comparable U.S. figure of 20.5 per 1,000 live births.

With every year there was an increase in hospital confinements, so that by 1953, more than half of the women were hospitalized. By 1974 only one or two mothers a month are having their babies at home, even though FNS is still willing to perform the service. This change has come about partly because of a shift in values and also because of a declining birth rate in the county due to increased birth control measures and the exodus of young people.

While dedicated organizations have been successful in administering comprehensive maternity care to the economically disadvantaged for three quarters of a century, the people they have been helping have gradually come to choose hospital deliveries. On the other hand, relatively recently a few upper and middle class families have begun to turn toward home births. These contemporary families are finding it gratifying, physically and psychologically. Coming full circle, out of the past there is a new way: Home birth for normal, healthy pregnancies is no longer a risky necessity but a remarkable and viable alternative.

One obvious question concerning home birth today is why do many people look back with nostalgia to a time fraught with risks and hardships in maternity? The answer is that those of us who believe in having our babies at home are not being either masochistic or foolish. Nobody wants it *exactly* the way it used to be. What many contemporary families do want is to preserve some of the old values that were lost with hospital deliveries. What we want is to take the *best* of the past. We cherish the shared moment, the intrinsic education for our other children, the personal dignity, the serenity. The joys of having a baby at home are exclusive of the past hardships. It is now possible to secure the best of both worlds—the past and the present.

Christmas Eve. It would be another Christmas with the sun shining brightly, and our first Christmas in seven years with the world at peace.

Yes, I would go to Shoal today, a good day to go since I would not have to ford Ole Man River—angry, snarling and boisterous and doing his best to reach "tide" before nightfall.

So with this thought in mind I saddled Kelpie and took off feeling that I had acted with the wisdom of Solomon. How very nice not to feel rushed. Everything was serene and peaceful except for Ole Man River, but I didn't have to cross him today.

After completing a five-mile ride I stopped at a cabin on Shoal Hill. I wanted to see the Moss family, but the Moss family had left these parts two weeks before. I was greeted by seven beautiful brown-eyed Smiths, ranging in age from two to ten years.

I went in the cabin and took up my position by a small fire in the grate which was trying desperately not to breathe its last. The mother of the seven youngsters was in bed in the back of the room with layer after layer of heavy quilts over her.

"Are you sick?" I asked.

"No ma'm. We just shoved in here last Tuesday on the edge of dark. I guess I did a little too much. You see I am expecting, but not yet. I'm wastin' awful."

With this bit of information I went into action, feeling rather bleak. I had no delivery bags; the husband was away; the river was up. But I soon found the "wastin'" was not so awful, and proceeded to ask the usual questions.

Then I said, "You are due to have your baby today."

She answered, "I can't get down today. Besides I have no miseries except a small misery in my back."

By this time I had decided Mr. Stork was arriving and on time. With the help of the ten-year-old I got the room arranged and the sickly fire going. I got out the small "emergency bag" we carry in our general nursing saddlebags for an emergency like this. All I could find in which to boil things up on the fire was the lid of a lard can, and I nearly spilled its contents in the ashes. By this time Mr. Stork was gathering speed and shortly came in with a fine eight-pound boy. At that moment father arrived. From the look of astonishment on his face I couldn't tell whether he thought I was something from Mars or just Santa Claus. When he had sufficiently recovered, I said to him, "I think your son would like a suit of clothes to put on in this kind of weather."

With a broad grin he set to work to find something. After much searching he came up with a red flannel petticoat—his son's first suit. It was warm at least, and appropriate to the Christmas season. It would have to suffice until I returned with one of the Frontier Nursing Service layettes.

At the edge of dark, which comes early in the mountains, I left a beautiful baby boy tucked cozily away in a suit of red, a happy father and mother, and seven little socks hanging over the fireplace, to make my way home through a gently falling snow. As Kelpie and I rode silently on we heard someone singing from a lonely cabin, "Silent Night, Holy Night."

MY CHRISTMAS EVE BABY, By Anna May January, R.N., C.M. Courtesy Frontier Nursing Service, Inc., QUARTERLY BULLETIN, Autumn, 1946.

139

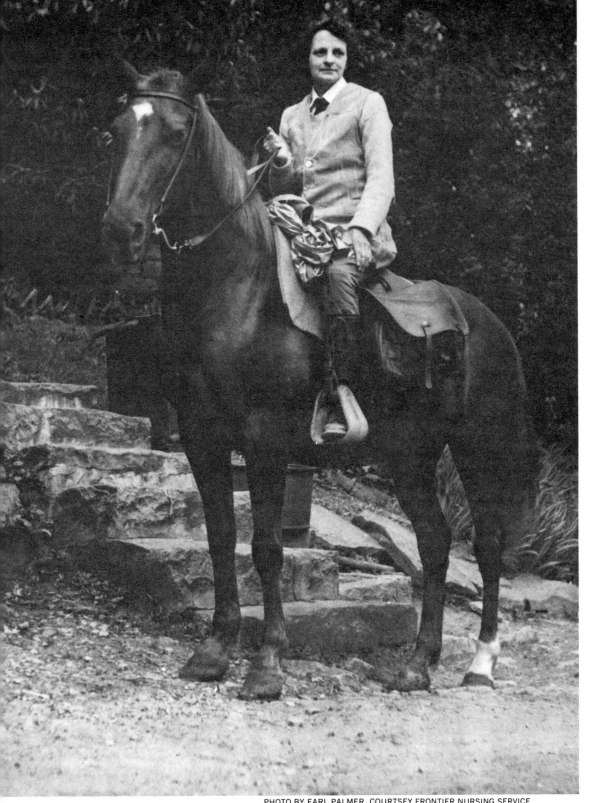

PHOTO BY EARL PALMER, COURTSEY FRONTIER NURSING SERVICE

Miss Anna May January of the Frontier Nursing Service on Cindy near Wendover, Ky., in the summer of 1950.

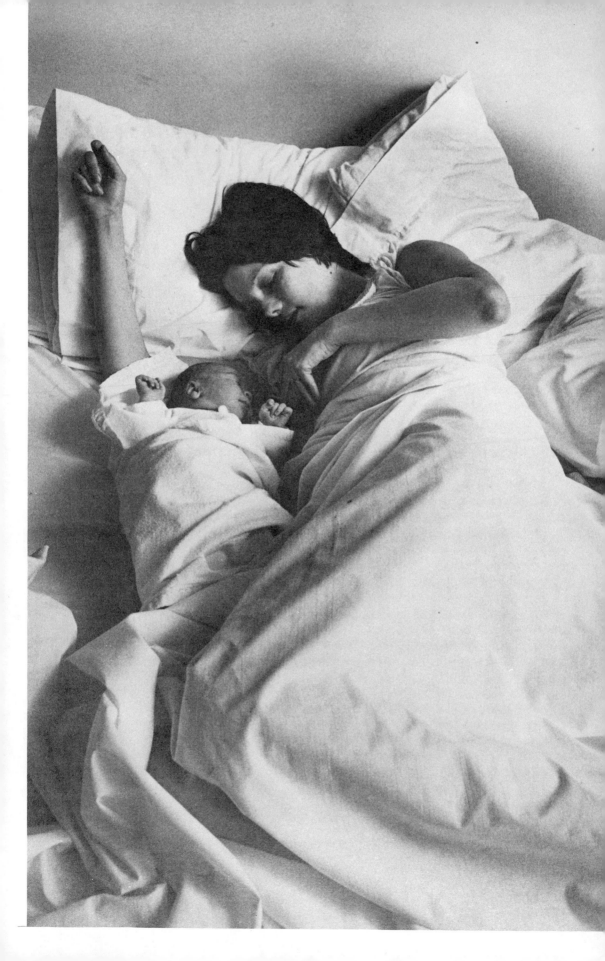

part 4

The Practical Dimension

BY TONYA BROOKS, PRESIDENT

The Association for Childbirth at Home, International

My decision to found the Association for Childbirth at Home came soon after the birth of my third child at home in 1972. For the entire summer preceding Cyrus' birth I searched high and low for a doctor to deliver me at home. My futility was shared by scores of other women whom I contacted in the search: "I don't know of anyone, but if you find someone please give me a call. I'd love to have my next baby at home!" Eventually my husband and I decided that if we were going to get our birth at home, we were going to have to educate ourselves to do it, because there were no professionals in the area willing to help. With the assistance of a woman who had delivered five of her own children at home, Cyrus was born in the quiet calm of our home in Arlington, Massachusetts, in September

of 1972. The birth was beautiful, my baby and I were fine, the entire family was together throughout the birth.

We were able to have our home birth, but only because of an incredible effort to make it happen. During our search for assistance we had discovered a huge unsatisfied demand for information and resources for birth at home. It was because of this need that I founded the Association for Childbirth at Home. (ACAH).

Since its founding in 1972 ACAH has grown enormously around the United States. We will soon have an ACAH group in every major city in the U.S. and groups in Canada, Australia, New Zealand, and Europe as well. This phenomenal growth has been spurred by a tremendous demand for information on home birth everywhere and can be attributed to an increasing consciousness of the physical, mental and spiritual implications of birth in general. Parents around the globe have begun to reassume responsibility for the birth of their own children.

ACAH is totally dedicated to helping parents and women take on the responsibility of decision making in where, how, and with whom they will give birth by getting them up-to-date medical and psychological information about birth. To do that we offer an intensive 6 week course (4 hours per week class time) called the ACAH Series to train parents in basic obstetrics. It is fundamental to our philosophy that parents must retain control of their own children's births—to simply delegate one's body over to hospital, doctor, or even midwife is dangerous and irresponsible.

In the first of the six weekly classes in the ACAH Series, called "Prerequisites for Safe Home Birth," parents and other interested people are taught high risk screening: medical prerequisites and

143

contraindications to home birth, the basic principles of good nutrition and the effects of a poor diet on pregnancy and birth, and how to participate in their own prenatal care.

We have found that the latter is particularly important since our experience with an ACAH survey in 1975 has shown that the level of prenatal care offered by doctors and clinics is totally inadequate for women giving birth at home. We have corrected this by teaching women how to use their own prenatal care charts to make certain that their doctors provided them with good quality prenatal care. Women are taught to find out what their normal pulse, blood pressure, blood type, and hemoglobin count are. They are taught about urine tests, pelvic measurement, and high risk screening. They are taught to find their own baby's heart rate. Along with data on good nutrition this training enables ACAH mothers to know precisely where problems may lie, what to do about them, and how to work intelligently with their doctors in prenatal care.

The "Prerequisites" class also covers the advantages of home birth, pro's and con's of home and hospital, and patients' rights: how to get the best birth possible if one has to go to a hospital. ACAH originally taught that women traded off the greater safety of the hospital for the psychological benefits of being at home. We taught that having the baby at home was worth the added risk because of the highly damaging psychological effects of standard hospital procedures, in particular the trauma of mother-baby separation after birth. Our own experience and the published research of others have since convinced us, however, that a low-risk mother puts herself in a higher risk category if she goes into a hospital, since she then exposes herself to iatrogenic (doctor or hospital induced) complica-

tions. By being in the hospital instead of the home, a mother risks a greater chance of infection for both herself and her baby. Amniotomy (rupturing the bag of waters) to insert the electrodes of an internal fetal heart monitor in the baby's head causes greater molding since the head rather than the amniotic sac takes the brunt of the pressure of cervical dilatation and forcing open of maternal tissues. And, of course, the standard lithotomy position (flat on the back) causes the mother to be pushing the baby *up* against gravity and can result in fetal distress through the baby's compressing the main arteries that feed oxygenated blood to the uterus.

The second class of our series is called "Management of the Normal Birth". It covers birth from the three points of view of the mother, the labor coach, and the midwife or other birth attendant. We teach the mechanism, anatomy, and physiology of each stage of labor and the sensations a woman can be expected to experience at each stage. Basic labor management is covered, each set of parents being taught to listen for the baby's heart beat, how to palpate the position of the baby, how to take maternal pulse and blood pressure. A midwive's perspective is taken in teaching perineal massage, procedures for catching the baby, suctioning of a newborn, etc. The necessary equipment and where to get it are also described. Parents are given the assignment to make their emergency backup plan which consists of having an adequately sized car with a tank full of gas, a telephone, known alternate routes to the nearest hospital, a private physician who will admit the woman to the hospital, and a pediatrician for the baby. Part of this plan is to know the admission rules and reputation of the hospital, ambulance services, and paramedics in the area. This plan is written up, brought to class to check for its thoroughness, and then posted by the parents' telephone at home. Lastly the class covers the husband's role in working with his wife to organize the home-birth team.

This class has been criticized as giving people enough knowledge to just "go out and do it themselves." We have found, however, that just as in the woman's self-help movement, the opposite thing has occurred: people became more aware of both their abilities and their limitations and more responsible in choosing their birth attendants.

The third class deals with the definable psychological issues of childbirth and to my knowledge these issues are covered so completely nowhere else. This class is perhaps the most important, because somewhere between 92 and 95 percent of us are going to have "normal" vaginal deliveries and healthy babies. For us birth is not a medical issue at all, but rather a psychological and spiritual experience that will directly affect the rest of our lives. In the seven years I have studied childbirth and infant-mother relationships, it has become clear that the psychological issues are universally important to women and are virtually ignored by the medical establishment. And yet fear, anxiety, emotional trauma, and upset can stop labor or prolong it significantly. For this reason ACAH emphasizes the husband's greatly expanded role at home. He controls the environment so that nothing upsets the laboring woman. This is easily done at home but virtually impossible in the hospital. Other psychological issues covered are how to keep one's pain threshold high and the relationship of pain threshold to fatigue, being overwhelmed and the resulting problems, diminishing or extinction of after birth ecstasy, diminuation of sibling rivalry, and sexuality related to childbirth. The latter includes diminished sexual desire, alterations of the woman's body and self-image by pregnancy and birth, and impact of episiotomies and circumcision.

The fourth class of the ACAH Series deals with obstetrical emergencies that are not predictable by prenatal care: what the symptoms are and what to do until one gets to the hospital. Both maternal emergencies such as hemorrhage, shock, and coma, and infant emergencies are defined and statistical chances of these things happening are discussed. All parents are taught how to recognize complications, how to give cardio-pulmonary resuscitation of the newborn, and how to handle hemorrhage until emergency assistance arrives or one arrives at the hospital. Obstetrics is not mysterious and lay people can understand it. However, there is no substitute for experience.

The fifth class is the result of three years of research into causes, cures, and controls of pain. We teach a breathing technique which is a variant of the Lamaze and other techniques but which differs sharply with the auto-hypnotic approach of psychoprophylaxis. It also covers prenatal exercises, massage, and reflexology. We have made breathing techniques work better consistently, helped women confront and manage difficult labors without drugs and keep their pain thresholds high without becoming overwhelmed.

The sixth class concerns the neonatal period of the first few days of the baby's life, the neonatal exam, what to look for when a doctor is needed, subtle signs of danger in newborns, nursing, and establishing good family-baby relationships. All parents are taught to determine the Apgar score of their new baby and common problems in the newborn.

To reach our goal of returning the control and responsibility of childbirth to the parents, we have expanded our levels of training and services tenfold in the last four years. We want women and parents to know we are totally dedicated to getting help to you in the form of courses and data as fast as we can train new ACAH leaders around the country and world.

Today there are a large number of groups teaching these basic principles in the ACAH Series to home birth parents. These groups are led by certified childbirth educators who have been trained in the ACAH Teacher Training Program which is now being offered on a nationwide basis (and in some foreign countries as well) to qualified applicants.

Our teacher training has a form consisting of three basic parts: (a) an extensive self-paced course in home-birth completed by the teacher trainee at home over a 1-6 month period depending on her background and the amount of time she spends on the course each week; (b) a Teacher Training Seminar which is offered to trainees in two forms: (1) monthly at the ACAH regional offices in Cerritos, California (near L.A.), and Kittery, Maine, (and soon to be offered in Seattle, Houston, St. Louis, and Miami) or (2) locally at the request of a group of trainees in an area relatively distant from the regional offices. Finally, (c) a certification examination is given to leader trainees to make certain they are ready to teach the ACAH Series to parents.

ACAH has recently begun a new level of training open to certified ACAH leaders called Advanced Leader Training. This program takes ACAH leaders with background and experience at home births and trains them as midwives. We developed this program to satisfy the tremendous need for trained help for parents and the desire of ACAH leaders to know more technical data on the birth process. This course is offered in ACAH training centers where it is clearly legal to teach midwifery.

In addition to the three levels of training discussed so far, ACAH offers several additional services to parents and others interested in home birth. We have an international referral service to doctors, midwives, and nurses who attend home births and to other groups that support home birth in one way or another. This referral service is currently being computerized in the Los Angeles area. Each ACAH leader offers a referral service of her own for the local area she serves. Each leader is also trained in prenatal screening and can give private counseling to women and parents to answer questions and help them plan their home births. ACAH has a speaker's bureau for university groups, service clubs, and other interested groups who would like to be informed about home birth, the home birth movement, and ACAH. We also offer intensive seminars on home birth to the public.

Finally we have an ongoing research project on the subject of home birth which involves a statistical questionnaire developed by ACAH. Anyone who has had a home birth is invited to participate in our study by writing for our questionnaire.

There is a charge for the ACAH Series and training programs. These funds enable us to pay our dedicated leaders and to support further development of ACAH and our research program.

We want people to know that we are totally committed to safe aesthetic birth experiences because we know better parent-child relationships and a better world will follow. We have found ACAH to be an excellent way to help and we are determined to help in any way that we can.

Anyone interested in our training programs and services may write to me personally at:

The Association for Childbirth at Home, International
P.O. Box 1219
Cerritos, California 90701

By Esther Herman
and Fran Ventre

H.O.M.E.

H.O.M.E. came to be in April, 1974, when a group of five women envisioned an educational organization devoted exclusively to helping couples in their quest for information and support for home birth. Over the years we had become aware that the phenomenon of modern home birth was gaining momentum and had attempted to help in various ways. As we met, it became obvious to us that a series of meetings directed toward the home birth couple was the answer, and we immediately set about to draft our purpose: "We are a group devoted to helping couples achieve the optimum experience of a safe home birth. We bring together those who have had home births, those who want home birth, professionals, and childbirth educators." What we could call our new group was the spontaneous and unanimous choice —H.O.M.E. Home Oriented Maternity Experience said it all.

H.O.M.E. has already become an incorporated non-profit educational organization with over 100 Leaders-in-training in several states and in Israel and 20 groups in operation. A master list of birth attendants has been compiled for nearly every state. Spreading knowledge of our group has produced an avalanche of mail, most of which is concerned with requesting names of birth attendants and other resource people in specific areas and the facts on how to have a home birth. Many have simply sent thanks for offering what they were unable to find elsewhere—the support and encouragement of sympathetic and experienced women.

All meetings are conducted by H.O.M.E. Leaders, who have been certified through an application process designed to assure competence in informing people about home birth. Interested persons, expectant parents, and their families and friends are all welcome to participate free of charge. There is a small membership fee for those who wish to join. Within the framework of five classes, those committed to home birth can prepare to take the ultimate responsibility for a safe and joyous experience.

First Meeting: Advantages of Home Birth

The positive aspects of home birth are emphasized, such as warmth, familiarity, comfort, freedom of choice, togetherness, and unimpaired bonding of the family. It is important to note that H.O.M.E. is pro home birth—not anti hospital birth. For those couples who may ultimately choose the hospital or may need to go to the hospital because of medical complications, we offer suggestions to help them make their hospital experience as "home-like" as possible.

We emphasize that in the home, the parents and baby can stay together, that bonding/imprinting can occur naturally and without interference, and that the baby can nurse as early and as frequently as it desires. We also discuss how siblings can be prepared for and involved in the home birth experience.

147

Second Meeting: Responsibilities, Equipment, and Procedures

In order to have a safe and healthy home birth, we feel the couple needs to take responsibility for the following: (1) excellent prenatal care, (2) above average nutrition, (3) excellent health, free of high risk indications for labor and delivery, (4) arrangements for competent medical assistance for the birth, (5) gathering supplies, and (6) intent to breastfeed the baby. We also recommend a full series of childbirth education, breastfeeding, and H.O.M.E. classes. Preparation and arrangements for the postpartum care of the mother are discussed at this time.

At this meeting we offer suggestions for setting up the birth area. We have available a list of birth attendants and pediatricians sympathetic to home birth and nursing. Those planning a home birth are encouraged to prepare also for the eventuality of a hospital birth by making a list of family-centered needs. Fulfillment of these needs, unless medically impossible, contributes to the health and well-being of both mother and infant as well as the father and the family unit as a whole.

Third Meeting: Psychological Issues

In a forum of open discussion, we cover such topics as expectations of the couple for their birth; attitudes of family, friends, and medical professionals toward home birth; psychobiological effects of the emotions on labor, on the baby, and on the couple; and postpartum adjustments of the couple and siblings. It is also important to discuss the possibility of hospitalization and what feelings may accompany such action. H.O.M.E. is sensitive to the disappointment that couples intent on home birth may experience. Because these psychological issues are complex and emotional, we feel that honest discussion helps home birth couples meet them in a postive way.

Fourth Meeting: Medical Considerations

In explaining the contraindications to home birth, we stress that almost all are predictable during good prenatal care and that excellent nutrition is the best insurance against many problems. We discuss what to do about unforeseen difficulties that may arise during labor, delivery, and postpartum. We also point out that many so-called difficulties of childbirth may actually be caused by interference with the natural process of labor and birth.

Fifth Meeting: Transition to Parenthood and Breastfeeding

This class is held to help parents in their new roles. Since we consider birth as the beginning of parenthood rather than an end in itself, we emphasize the importance of the postpartum period. In this meeting we give a thorough overview of breastfeeding, its health implications to mother and baby, and the need for immediate and frequent nursing after birth. We also discuss possible early problems and how they can be handled or avoided. We talk about the realities of the needs of newborns and try to help couples visualize the unyielding character of their new responsibility.

Looking to the future, H.O.M.E. hopes to become a clearinghouse for various research and study projects. Accurate current statistics on home birth are needed. We believe that carefully controlled studies will show that home birth is safer than hospital birth for the low risk woman. In addition, we intend to implement programs for professional midwives, such as are currently operating in England and the Netherlands. Helping the medical establishment to understand and become sensitive to the needs of the home birth couple is another goal. As consumer advocates, we will work to change and update antiquated laws to meet the current status of home births in this country.

ORGANIZATIONS THAT HELP

Home Birth
American College of Home Obstetrics
664 North Michigan Avenue, Suite 600
Chicago, Illinois 60611

Maternity Center of El Paso
P.O. Box 3063, Station A
El Paso, Texas 79923

Maternity Center Associates, Ltd.
5415 Cedar Lane, Suite 208A
Bethesda, Maryland 20014

National Association of Parents and Professionals for
    Safe Alternatives in Childbirth (NAPSAC)
David and Lee Stewart
P.O. Box 1307
Chapel Hill, North Carolina 27514

Prepared Childbirth
American Society for Psychoprophylaxis in Obstetrics (A.S.P.O.)
National Headquarters
1523 L Street, N.W. Room 105
Washington, D.C. 20005

Holistic Childbirth Institute
1627 Tenth Avenue
San Francisco, California 94122

International Childbirth Education Association
P.O. Box 5852
Milwaukee, Wisconsin 53220

Breastfeeding
La Leche League International, Inc.
9616 Minneapolis Avenue
Franklin Park, Illinois 60131

$5.95

THE HOME BIRTH BOOK

BY CHARLOTTE AND FRED WARD
INTRODUCTION BY ASHLEY MONTAGU, Ph.D.

Home birth is not just a counter-culture phenomenon, but rather a loving family experience that allows immediate bonding between mother and child. THE HOME BIRTH BOOK should be read by anyone considering having a baby at home, or for anyone interested in exploring experiences which humanize their lives in an increasingly mechanized society. It explores the home birth alternative in all its dimensions: personal, medical, psychological, sociological, and historical.

Here is what reviewers have said about the book:

". . . it may well serve as a basic reference on an alternative to hospital deliveries . . . The photography of the many home births . . . captures the concern and the sharing of a joyously happy, meaningful experience." *The Journal of Primal Therapy*

". . . the photographs by Fred Ward . . . are probably the best seen in any childbirth book to date." *Bookmarks*

". . . informative and well presented . . . obviously a labor of love, and this love shines through in the text and the lovely photographs." *La Leche News*

The Wards are the parents of three children, two of whom were born at home. Charlotte has long been active in La Leche League. Fred is a photo-journalist whose work has appeared in *Time, Newsweek, Life, National Geographic,* and many other publications.

A Doubleday Dolphin Book
COVER PHOTOGRAPH BY FRED WARD
COVER DESIGN BY JOSEPH MERLO

ISBN: 0-385-12559-3

Date Due

NOV 2 0 1978

NOV

MAR 2 8 1979

MAY 0

JUL 2 5 19

AUG 2 2 1979

NOV 0 7 1979

NOV 2 8 1979

MAR 1 7 1980

APR 1 6 1980

MAY 0 7 1980

JUL 1 0 1980

MAR 2 5 1981

MAR 2 8 1984

APR 2 5 1984

NOV

APR 2 9 19

JUL 1 5 1981T

DEC 0 2 1981

MAR 1 7 1982

APR 1

JUN 0 2 1982

NOV 0

OCT 2

APR 2 7

APR 1 8 1994

APR 1 9 2000

APR 1 8

APR 0 1

MAY 0 1

MAR 3 0 1988

MAY 1 3 1993

MAY 0 5 1998

MAY 0 9 702

DRAKE MEMORIAL LIBRARY

E COLLEGE AT BROCKPORT

BRODART, INC

Cat No 23 233

PRINTED IN U.S.A.   CAT. NO. 24 161

BRO DART